D0931510

Options for School Health

Meeting Community Needs

"Presentation of this volume was assisted by a grant from The Robert Wood Johnson Foundation, Princeton, New Jersey. The opinions, conclusions, and proposals in the text are those of the author(s) and do not necessarily represent the views of The Robert Wood Johnson Foundation."

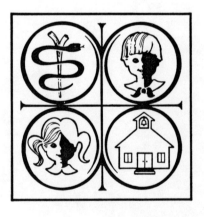

Options for School Health

Options for School Health

Meeting Community Needs

Philip R. Nader, M.D.
Editor

In Collaboration with:
John G. Bruhn, Ph.D.
Elizabeth Bryan, M.D.
Guy S. Parcel, Ph.D.
James Williams, M.S.W.

ASPEN SYSTEMS CORPORATION
GERMANTOWN, MARYLAND
1978

Library of Congress Cataloging in Publication Data

Main entry under title:

Options for school health.

Includes index.
1. School hygiene. I. Nader, Philip R.
LB3405.C67   371.7   78-9628
ISBN: 0-89443-038-6

Library of Congress Catalog Card Number: 78-9628
ISBN: 0-89443-038-6

Printed in the United States of America

1 2 3 4 5

Table of Contents

Contributors to This Volume

Editor:

Philip R. Nader, M.D.
Associate Professor of Pediatrics and
   Psychiatry and Behavioral Sciences
Director, School Health Programs
The University of Texas Medical Branch
Galveston, Texas 77550

In collaboration with:

John G. Bruhn, Ph.D.
Associate Dean for Community Affairs
The University of Texas Medical Branch
Galveston, Texas 77550

Elizabeth Bryan, M.D.
School Physician
Edmonds School District
Edmonds, Washington 98020

Guy S. Parcel, Ph.D.
Assistant Professor of Pediatrics and
   Preventive Medicine & Community Health
Health Educator, School Health Programs
The University of Texas Medical Branch
Galveston, Texas 77550

James Williams, M.S.W.
Community Organization Specialist and
  Coordinator of Educational Planning
  Office of the Dean of Medicine
The University of Texas Medical Branch
Galveston, Texas 77550

Contributing Editors:

Susan Gilman, M.S.
Evaluator
School Health Programs
The University of Texas Medical Branch
Galveston, Texas 77550

Christine Grant, M.B.A.
Program Officer
The Robert Wood Johnson Foundation
Princeton, New Jersey 08540

Katherine P. Messenger, M.C.P.
Lecturer in Child Health
Harvard School of Public Health
Boston, Massachusetts 02115

Philip J. Porter, M.D.
Director, Department of Pediatrics
The Cambridge Hospital
Cambridge, Massachusetts 02139

Mildred C. Williamson, R.N.
Coordinator of Health Services
The Galveston Independent School District
Galveston, Texas 77550

Preface

*The society we imagine would be one that put children first, not
last, that saw the development of a vital, resourceful, caring,
moral generation of Americans as the nation's highest
priority—All Our Children,* by Kenneth Keniston and The Car-
negie Council on Children. Harcourt, Brace, Jovanovich 1977.

In this era of "You can't get there from here," I find this a refreshing
book. It is straightforward in its premise that every child should have a
medical home, and that schools can contribute towards implementation
of this goal.

Like access to education, there is no Constitutional guarantee to access
to health care, but there is in this country an unwritten presumption that
the way to safeguard the health and welfare of our population is to
guarantee certain basic services. How this is accomplished varies enor-
mously from state to state, community to community. Policy making in
education, health and welfare is the responsibility of the localities, but
the state legislature holds ultimate control. In between, there are a host
of professional people who are trying to influence policy—the governor,
and his appointees to head state departments of health, education and
welfare; professional staff in these agencies; citizens on state boards;
county and city leaders; school superintendents; principals; teachers;
physicians; dentists; nurses; local board members; and, of course, the
children and their families acting on their behalf.

The authors accept the situation's complexity and proceed to propose
ways to work with the system.

The schools are one of a number of settings for providing health care to children. In many communities, the schools may be a screening and referral point. In other communities, they may be the logical place to provide services beyond screening. Either way, according to the authors of this book, the underlying issue in assuring children access to health care is the need for a partnership between the education and the health care worlds. worlds.

The book is a practical manual. The material in its chapters grew out of a meeting in which the authors and others were participants. One intriguing chapter reports how participants returned home from the meeting to implement what they had learned, and were successful in doing so.

While communities may take different approaches to guaranteeing the health and well-being of the children, the schools have an educational role that needs to be reviewed. Health as subject matter has never been among the basics. No curriculum supervisor would place it alongside mathematics, reading, and writing. I ask, Why Not? Children are naturally curious about themselves, their bodies and their minds. They often are not only curious, but concerned and worried. The intensity of their interest provides a "teachable moment," and when children present a medical or dental problem, they are possibly in that moment. What schools can address is how to capture that moment, how to provide children with a fair and reasonable understanding of their physical and emotional make up, and how to help them assume responsibility for monitoring their state of health. If the schools acknowledged at least that goal, we would have made a step forward in educating our young to cope with life.

Margaret E. Mahoney
Vice President
The Robert Wood Johnson Foundation

Acknowledgment

The contributions of Marilyn Thompson, the Technical Editor, and Judi Godwin and Mary Anne Mabry, typists, are gratefully acknowledged.

Introduction

Philip R. Nader, M.D.

WHY OPTIONS FOR SCHOOL HEALTH?

School health means different things to different people, and it varies from one community to the next. It can mean only bandages and first aid, or the only way in which children receive health care and health education so they can derive the most benefit from their educational experience, or a method of guaranteeing access to health care providers for all children in a community. Today, some school health "programs" include educational activities, whereas other school health "services" are strictly outside the educational program and excluded from any involvement in student curriculum.

Regardless of which one is chosen, it is important for each community to arrive at a definition of school health that will work in that community. This need is immediate. Financial constraints on education are increasing, along with parallel increases in the costs of and demand for comprehensive health services. For too long, health services in schools have been approached, or neglected, on the basis that such services are "good" and "supplemental," but not of practical importance.

Today real problems face all schools which are required to better integrate health and educational services. New mandatory special education laws require that public schools serve handicapped persons ages 3 to 21 years. A child who has to have his throat stroked to swallow food is not a routine student for most teachers. Education of the handicapped will require health personnel to be involved intimately with school personnel. For services to be provided to the many children handicapped by neurologic and psychological problems, medical and health evaluations and follow-up are necessary.

One of the crises facing health care is access to and appropriate utilization of health care resources. Competent patients/consumers will know how to explore and interpret their own physical and emotional feelings, assess the degree of need for assistance, and obtain the help they need. Life skills such as these have long been assigned to the school to teach. The challenge to health education includes the following questions: How can people learn to become responsible for their own health/illness needs? How can young children learn these skills? Are current school health education programs really addressing these issues?

The concept of options for school health, therefore, implies that each community has different needs and resources that dictate different options for the scope and nature of the school health program. The needs and resources of urban and suburban areas differ and, therefore, demand unique solutions. The options developed as best for any community will succeed if they take into account the local characteristics of that community: the families and children, the school personnel and policies, and the providers of health care.

PURPOSE

This book is for school personnel and health care providers on the front line. It is intended to be a source book for them, many of whom already know the "what" of school health but share the frustration of discovering the "how" of achieving the full potential impact of school health programs. The book recognizes that "education" of children for life skills is too important a task to be left to educators alone, and that "promoting the health" of children is too important to be left to health care providers alone. Also included is an appreciation of the rights and responsibilities of individuals and families to be active, free agents in seeking and obtaining health care and health promotion services.

CONTENT

The content of this book can be applied to any individual community developing a model or framework for school health. As a prerequisite to model building, the data available on the nature of the bond between the health and the education of young children will be reviewed. Then, a rationale behind planning for restructuring, changing, or beginning school health programs based on the nature of the community will be given. The rationale will be illustrated with concrete examples of program activities and services.

Actual examples of model building are presented, drawn from community case studies presented at a National Conference on School Health held at The University of Texas Medical Branch at Galveston in June 1976 and attended by 200 educators, health professionals, laymen, and representatives of national organizations related to child health and education. Two distinct, successful models of school health programs—one operating largely within the educational system, the other largely within the health system—will be described. The descriptions will include the steps that participants took to overcome some of the traditional barriers that often impede cooperative working efforts.

Finally, implementing specific school health program outcomes and objectives will be described, along with currently known options for budgeting and financing of school health programs.

DOING A NEW THING—PLANNING FOR CHANGE

It is necessary to recognize that there are goals that are more important than the activities carried out traditionally in our own bailiwicks. We will develop a basis for our activities that recognizes each of our systems as a component of a larger system, the human community. The "new thing" in school health then becomes how to use a technology of organizational change and development. The goals of change should help us to identify avenues of change that exist in our respective systems and to harness them to this issue; to create, if necessary, new structures of organizational cooperation; and to locate and focus all the necessary resources in our systems to make it all possible.

From this point of view, the resources of a community are seen not as a severely limited commodity for which there is already too much competition, but as an unlimited potential already present in the strengths of the individuals, families, groups, and institutions of the whole community. The greatest danger for the future of school health will not be in planning too big, but—with timidity—in thinking too small.

Chapter 1

Competence: The Outcome of Health and Education

Philip R. Nader, M.D., and
Guy S. Parcel, Ph.D.

Health care is not equivalent to health. Education is not the same as learning. Health and learning must be defined by more than the current performance of the institutions that claim to serve these ends.[1] "Competence...[implies] intelligence in the broadest sense, operative intelligence, 'knowing how' rather than simply 'knowing that.' For competence implies action, changing the environment as well as adapting to the environment."[2]

Schools are institutions charged with endowing children with life skills to make them competent, contributing individuals in society. Yet, many children learn failure and frustration in school rather than self-confidence. Schools continue to identify increasing numbers of children as suffering from some sort of educational or learning problem; and, in addition to that burden, public schools are being asked to be responsible for the socialization and education of handicapped persons. These are among the recent challenges to schools as they attempt to prepare children with life skills.

At the same time, hundreds of thousands of Americans die prematurely from diseases or conditions that are lethal because of the individual's lack of competence in managing his/her life style as it pertains to his/her health. Examples of such deaths in 1973 include 757,075 from heart disease, 115,821 from accidents, 33,350 from cirrhosis of the liver, 25,118 from suicide, 20,465 from homicide, and 7,428 from hypertension.[3] The challenge to health care institutions is to prevent such deaths by educating people to be more competent in their decision making about their own health.

It is impossible to separate the effects of health on education from those of education on health. Few would deny that a child's potential to become competent is influenced by many health factors—genetic, nutritional, physical, psychological, and social. One's health status is a determinant of competence in education, and educational experiences should provide the skills to be a competent, self-directed, and appropriate user of health services.

Truly responsive school health programs should promote competence in children by developing activities that are designed to overcome any blocks to each child's attainment of competence. In other words, school health programs should ask: what circumstances can we identify that impede a child's ability to become competent? The answers to this question should point the way toward developing school health programs that exist not merely because "we've always had school health" or that "principals and parents expect it."

HEALTH FACTORS INFLUENCING LEARNING

Mortality Rates

Infant mortality rates have declined from 1964 to 1974 from 24.8 to 16.5 deaths per 1,000 live births in the first year of life.[4] The majority of these deaths occur during the first month. Highest rates occur in lower socioeconomic and nonwhite populations. Although more children are surviving, many who do live suffer insults of prematurity and perinatal stress resulting in sequelae important to their later development.

Mortality rates among school-age children (5 to 14 years) in 1973 were (per 100,000 population): motor vehicle, 10.6; all other accidents, 10.2; malignant neoplasms, 5.4; congenital anomalies, 2.2; influenza and pneumonia, 1.4; homicide, 1.1; and all others, 2.7. Mortality rates for both accidents and infectious diseases are much higher for minority and poor school-age children than for other children in our country.

With deaths in infants and children decreasing, the number of children to be educated could increase—if the declining birth rate levels off. Regardless of the total number, however, the proportion of potentially handicapped children is certain to increase.

The disproportionate toll among lower socioeconomic school-age children from accidents (as well as infectious diseases) should alert planners of school health programs to the need for accident prevention among certain populations. For example, one of the leading causes of injury and death to small children is automobile accidents. Proper restraints or seat belts have been demonstrated to reduce disability from auto accidents significantly, but nothing tried so far has made any great change in the use of restraints by children. Perhaps schools are in the best position to influence the largest number of people to work toward change. Likewise, respiratory or other infectious illnesses should not be treated lightly among school populations with negative environmental influences such as poverty, overcrowding, undernutrition, or lack of ready access to health care resources.

Acute Morbidity

Recent information from the National Health Survey of 1973-1974 shows that acute illnesses (mostly respiratory) and injuries account for most of the restricted activity, missed school days, and doctor or hospital visits among the child population, 6 to 16 years of age.[5] Again, poor children are more likely to suffer transient disability than children from affluent homes, yet they are less likely to seek or receive health care. If one goal of school health programs is to limit absenteeism, educators will need to initiate investigative and follow-up activities designed to solve that problem and return the child to school. Higher level and more skilled assessment of common illnesses such as respiratory diseases (upper respiratory infections, strep throat, ear infection) by school health personnel should lead to their identification and resolution sooner and, thus, to fewer missed school days.

Chronic Morbidity

Chronic illness or the long-term effects of perinatal problems have an obvious impact on the ability of children to function optimally in school and in life. H. Knobloch and B. Pasamanich drew associations between brain damage and mental retardation and found them to be correlated with low birth weight, lower socioeconomic and minority group status, and lack of access to perinatal care.[6] Among 96 small-for-date newborns, one-fourth had speech defects, and 50 percent of the boys and 36 percent of the girls had poor school performance on follow-up.[7]

Less dramatic insults, including viral infections and transient starvation, have also been associated with later deficits in learning performance.[8,9] Malnutrition, both prenatal and postnatal, has been shown to decrease the number of brain cells. "Prolonged malnutrition, particularly if it occurs before five years of age, may lastingly affect learning ability, body growth, rate of maturation, as well as ultimate size and productivity."[10] Roughly one-fourth of all U.S. children live in families

3

whose income falls below the minimum considered necessary for adequate nutrition.[11] In 1972 only one-third of poverty-level children attending public school participated in school lunch programs.[12] How active is the school health program in ensuring access to food stamp and subsidy lunch and breakfast programs for children and families in need of this support? What specific activities relate to identification and follow-up of such families?

Other chronic conditions have either a direct or an indirect bearing on the child's acquisition of skills. School personnel long have recognized the need for screening for sensory defects, such as vision and hearing; but the benefit of screening is often lost because of poor follow-up or a lack of access to health care. School health programs need to address more attention to procedures designed to ensure that treatment or correction will be sought for all identified defects. Delays can result in needless classroom problems and learning handicaps that are often difficult to overcome during later years.

School-related behavioral, psychosomatic, learning, and adjustment problems are being identified more often as the most common concern of parents of school-age children.[13] Large numbers of children are on psychoactive drugs.[14] How can the school health program assist with regular assessments and follow-up activities for these children? Is academic improvement regularly monitored for children on medication, or only reports of classroom behavior? What in-service programs for teachers are held to improve their own understanding and management skills of such a child's behavior?

Discipline problems, child abuse, and delinquency are also barriers to learning, sometimes with long-lasting impact on children. What policies and programs have school health programs initiated or collaborated in with others in these areas? An estimated nine million Americans are alcoholics or problem drinkers.[15] Drinking among teen-agers is now nearly universal; 36 percent of high school students report getting drunk at least four times a year.[16] What is the school health program doing about this problem?

Chronic physical or medical conditions are likely to have an adverse affect on a child's general functioning in school and on the individual's ability to learn to manage his or her problem successfully. For example, a visible deformity or cosmetic defect might instill fear in peers or teachers—or cause outright rejection. An invisible defect, such as that causing seizures or diabetes, can likewise inspire fear that an unannounced crisis will occur in class. A constant atmosphere of dread can result—hardly conducive to a healthy self-concept or feelings of adequacy in the affected student. Most school health programs include a per-

4

functory acknowledgment to teachers of the existence of a student's medical condition that is likely to cause a problem in the classroom. How many also try to determine any deficits in the knowledge or attitude of students or teachers that will be detrimental to the affected student's best handling of the handicap? What is then done to modify these deficits?

EDUCATIONAL FACTORS INFLUENCING HEALTH

We have so far been considering those health factors that impinge on education. What about the other side of the coin, the influence of education upon health? There are fewer data, but more hope, on this side of the issue. Educating children about health is not a new concept for schools in the United States. Some form of instruction about health and safety has been a traditional part of most elementary and secondary schools for more than 30 years. Despite this long experience with health instruction in the schools, we know almost nothing about its long-term effects on health behavior or health status.

In 1964 the report of the first phase of the School Health Education (SHE) study identified several problems in school health education: omission or neglect of certain areas of health content, unnecessary repetition of learning experiences in other areas, lack of a logical basis for the placement of health education opportunities at various grade levels, and lack of a planned curriculum.[17]

The second phase of the SHE study attempted to overcome some of these problems by offering a framework for curriculum development in health education.[18] Several states and local school districts adopted the conceptual approach to curriculum design in health education that was recommended by the SHE study. The report of the President's Committee on Health Education published in 1973, however, indicated that many of the problems with school health education had not improved since 1964. "Our findings are that school health education in most primary and secondary schools either is not provided at all, or loses its proper emphasis because of the way it is tacked onto another subject such as physical education or biology, assigned to teachers whose interests and qualifications lie elsewhere."[19] The report further offers the following explanations for the inadequacies in school health education:

Antiquated laws, indifferent parents, unaggressive school boards, teachers poorly equipped to handle the subject, lack of leadership from government or the public, lack of funds, lack of research, lack of evaluation—all of those hobble a comprehensive program that could provide the nation's 55 million school children (one-fourth of the entire population) with adequate health education of an interesting, pertinent and objective nature.[20]

Even though the report is critical of school health education in general, the problems it refers to are not universal; and many school districts have made sincere efforts to develop effective health education programs. New approaches and materials and improved training are being tried in various communities and institutions throughout the country. Some school health education programs have been able to document changes in knowledge and attitudes, but we still do not know the overall effects of education on health status or health behavior.

The absence of data to demonstrate a relationship between learning about health in the schools and improved health behavior does not suggest the elimination of school health education. We have had enough experience to identify some approaches that are ineffective—ones that are neither interesting to the students nor offer them ways of applying learning to their daily living. For example, we know that boring lectures, didactic presentations of material, overuse of films, fear tactics, poorly prepared teachers, content inappropriate for age level, repetition of content at every grade level, and an absence of learning directed toward behavior objectives are ineffective educational methods. There is no need to continue programs that have the foregoing characteristics. In contrast, however, we know from the educational literature that children are more likely to learn and be interested if the learning experiences involve their active participation, if the content is related to real life experiences, if they can apply what they are learning while they are learning it, if content is appropriate for age level and student needs, and if teachers and students are working toward specified behavioral objectives (they know what they are expected to be able to do as a result of the learning activities). There *is* a need to develop programs that have these characteristics.

In addition to programs designed according to these sound educational principles, what we need is both a broadening and a narrowing of focus for school health education. A broadening in terms of how we conceptualize health, and a narrowing of what we can reasonably expect to accomplish through learning activities in the school. The title of this chapter implies that health means more than physical well-being: learning about health means more than learning about our needs for physical care and the structure and functioning of the body. Health education must also include an understanding of personal, social, and emotional needs; relationships with other people; coping with environmental stress; and solving problems.

A broad concept of health makes it even more critical for school health education programs to be more defined in what they intend to accomplish. One of the problems that has been observed with an expanding concept of health is that school programs have become so general, all-inclusive, and "comprehensive" that no one is really sure what the expected outcomes of the program are. Although data from school health programs are not available to develop a more exact definition of health education, data are accumulating from health education programs outside the school setting. Lawrence Green has reviewed the research on health education and has derived from it some recommendations to make educational programs more specific. He identifies three areas in which goals can be specified: immediate versus intermediate versus ultimate goals.[21]

Immediate Goals

According to L.W. Green, the immediate goals are changes in three types of factors (he calls them predisposing, enabling, and reinforcing factors) that are known or expected to be causally related to the health behavior in question. Based on a review of the literature, the following general components of health education programs are suggested as the most effective:

1. communication methods directed at the consumers (school children or parents) and the general public are most effective in achieving changes in *predisposing factors* such as knowledge, attitudes, beliefs, and norms;
2. community organization methods directed at other agencies and institutions are generally most effective in achieving changes in the *enabling factors,* which facilitate or inhibit health practices, such as availability and accessibility of services, referral mechanisms, third-party payment mechanisms, clinic hours, etc.;
3. staff development methods directed at the health providers and other personnel who interact with the consumers are most effective in achieving changes in the *reinforcing factors,* such as the attitudes and actions of clinic personnel toward walk-in patients, the rewards and punishments that parents and teachers provide children in response to health actions, or that employers provide employees in response to safety practices.[22]

A voluntary screening program in the schools, such as scoliosis screening, is an example of a health education program designed to meet immediate goals. An awareness of the screening program, a belief that the screening is important and valuable, and a willingness to participate can be considered *predisposing factors*. Effective communication and interaction with children and parents need to be planned to influence each of the three predisposing factors.

Enabling factors are those that facilitate student involvement in the screening, such as easy access to the screening, making students feel comfortable with the process, and conducting the screening in an efficient and organized manner. Removing possible barriers to the involvement of students constitutes an enabling factor. For example, requiring signed parental permission for screening might be an unnecessary barrier, preventing students from participating. The education program can attempt to overcome this barrier with an effort to achieve agreement among parents, health care providers, and school administrators to work toward students being able to give permission for their participation without the signed consent of parents.

Reinforcing factors in the educational program are, for example, preparing teachers, parents, school nurses, and health care providers to help the students feel good about participating in the screening—that their decision to participate is one way they can take positive action for their own health care.

As can be seen in this example, an educational program directed toward immediate goals involves more than providing information about health or a particular health problem (scoliosis). The program is more likely to be effective if it addresses changes in the predisposing, enabling, and reinforcing factors.

Intermediate Goals

The intermediate goals of health education are the behaviors expected to result if the immediate goals are accomplished.[23] Most school health education programs fall short in specifying and in evaluating behavior that is expected to result from the health instruction. Rarely is an investigation made to determine if students can do what is expected. The behavior that should result from the education should be specified in the planning phase. In the scoliosis screening program, for example, the expected behaviors might include: student participation in the screening; for those who are found to have scoliosis, a follow-through on referral to medical evaluation; and for those requiring treatment, a follow-through with treatment procedures.

Ultimate Goals

According to Green, the ultimate goals of health education programs consist of reductions in mortality, morbidity, and disability.[24] With a specific problem, such as scoliosis, it is easier to define ultimate goals. It is possible to determine how many cases of scoliosis can be prevented from progressing to the point that they require surgery and to what extent possible disability is prevented. It is also possible to measure reduction in morbidity for such things as sexually transmitted diseases, pregnancy, dental disease, and accidents.

Health education is not limited, however, to physical diseases or disorders. Social and emotional health deserve as much attention, even though it is more difficult to define the ultimate goals. Evaluation is especially difficult because the outcomes are often remote from the actual time period that learning activities are conducted. Also, short-term intervention is often not enough to produce a change, so long-range programs are necessary. In these areas, health education goals should include: assisting in developing the competencies to cope with stress, getting along with others, adapting to or changing one's environment, and utilizing resources for dealing with specific health-related problems.

METHODS OF IMPROVING HEALTH EDUCATION

Skills Approach to Health Education

We have reached a period when the promotion of health is dependent more on what individuals can learn to do for themselves than on what others do for them. The critical task for educators and health professionals is to plan for and provide children with learning experiences that will assist them in developing competencies. If one is competent, one is able to assume responsibility for one's own health, which includes self-directing behavior and being able to make appropriate use of available health resources.

Skills form the building blocks of competence. To reach a level of competence, children need to learn skills to enable them to make decisions about their health. J. Elliott and K. J. Connolly offer the following definition of a skill:

> It refers to the organization of actions into a purposeful plan which is executed with economy. Even in the case of such relatively imprecise concepts as "social skills," the essence of the skill lies in the ability to achieve a goal. . . . A broad descrip-

tion of skill therefore is "an ability to achieve defined goals with an efficiency beyond that of the inexperienced person."[25]

This definition implies that the learning of skills requires the opportunity to gain experience in using the skills. Teaching should allow the individual to practice using the constituents of the skill in as many contexts as possible. Connolly and J. S. Bruner point out further that competence involves more than cognition.

> ... one should equally well note the importance of nonspecific "emotional" skills: self-confidence is a good example of one such. One does not usually characterize it as a "skill" but as a trait or an attitude toward oneself. Yet it is a skill as well, for it involves learning that one can do things with a certain likelihood of success and moreover, with a fair likelihood of being able to run the course again should one fail.[26]

Competence, then, implies not only cognitive skills but also affective skills. As we look at various forms of health and illness behavior, it is not difficult to see that we are dealing with issues very different from other areas of learning such as language, mathematics, and motor performance. Affective skills take on central importance in dealing with health-related behaviors. For example, the decision of a junior high school student to smoke is probably related more to skills of self-understanding, dealing with peer pressure, and decision making than the skill of understanding the dangers and risks of smoking.

C. E. Lewis and M. A. Lewis have developed a model for health behavior that emphasizes the integration of both cognitive and social learning.[27] The social variables that explain adult utilization of health services also explain child utilization of school health services. Knowledge and past and present experiences are not sufficient by themselves to explain children's health behavior. Having information, or even developing correct concepts of health and illness, does not necessarily result in competent behavior. Individuals need to go beyond knowing and understanding to application within the context of daily living. For example, we can effectively teach children the importance of selecting food from the four food groups; but unless we also help the child to translate this knowledge into appropriate patterns of nutritional behavior we have failed in our health education efforts. There is a need to develop approaches to health education curriculum design that will more effectively integrate conceptual learning and social learning. The suggested skills approach to health education is an attempt to move in that direction.

The skills approach requires identification of skills, consideration of content and process necessary to develop the identified skills, and provision of opportunities to practice these skills. A general skill such as the ability to communicate feelings can apply to a specific desired behavioral outcome. For example, a health education activity for kindergarten children could be directed toward the outcome: children will be able to tell adults the different feelings they have when they think they might be sick. The content (what children need to learn) and the process (how they will learn) are then designed to be incorporated into the kindergarten curriculum to promote the development of this specific skill.

J. D. Swisher has outlined four general skill areas and has indicated the limited research that shows a relationship of these skills to health behavior.[28] General skill areas include:

1. personal skills—those internal perceptions (for example, self-concepts) and skills (for example, decision making) that are necessary for personal satisfaction with life;
2. interpersonal skills—those skills in relationships (for example, acceptance of others and listening) that are necessary for successful functioning in society;
3. extrapersonal skills—those skills that allow the individual to participate fully in society to the extent that its institutions serve the individual's needs (for example, having the ability to seek and obtain services within existing health care systems); and
4. health problem skills—those skills or perceptions that allow the individual to cope effectively with various health problems.

The specific skills to be identified in each of these four areas will be dependent on the characteristics of the learner population. Some skills, such as self-confidence, could be considered important to all. The emphasis placed on the learning activities related to this skill, however, will depend on present levels of attainment. The Division of Health, Safety, and Physical Education of the North Carolina Department of Public Instruction has published a series of curriculum guides titled "Life Skills for Health" that can provide additional examples of specific skills applied to health behavior.[29]

Curriculum Planning

Typical curriculum planning in health education has centered on organizing content into subject or topic areas. This approach focuses attention on what the student needs to know rather than what the student needs to be able to do. The skills approach suggests, first, that the developmental characteristics and health needs of a specific age group should be identified. Then planning should focus on what skills are needed and can be learned by children at a particular age. Content to be learned is not determined until the skills have been specified, and then the content is related directly to the learning of the skills.

The process, how children learn, should be as experiential as possible. Younger children, especially, are more likely to develop skills if the learning process involves applied practice. For example, children are more likely to learn decision-making skills in selecting healthy foods if they learn through the actual experience of selecting foods and receive social reinforcement for selecting the appropriate foods.

The final step in skill development is practice. In the classroom, children usually get plenty of practice in mathematics, language, and reading; but few classroom teachers provide the opportunity to practice health skills. The student needs to have the opportunity to practice the skill within different contexts. Within the classroom setting, simulated situations can provide an opportunity for practice; role playing and educational games are frequently used for this purpose. The classroom is limited, however, in its ability to offer real-life practice of skills. This is the point at which health education activities need to be extended outside the confines of the schoolroom.

A close relationship between classroom health education and school health services provides a natural opportunity for practice and the reinforcement of health-related skills. For example, one of the skills for third graders might be a differential utilization of health services—knowing when it is appropriate to seek health services and being able to seek the appropriate service. Classroom activities could be used to teach the content related to this skill. Then the children could practice by being allowed to make their own decisions as to when to see the school nurse or when to call their doctor. In the classroom, they can talk about their experiences and share feelings as well as any new knowledge that might have been gained through the practice experiences.

The involvement of parents is an additional important source of enhancing practice of skills, for two reasons: it assists the parents in supporting the practice and reinforcement of skills their children are learning, and it assists parents in developing skills that will enable them to be more competent as parents. Also, efforts should be made to involve health care providers in the planning of school health education programs and curricula. A close relationship between school personnel and community health personnel is important to increase the possibility that children will have the opportunity to apply their skills within the health care delivery system.

Planning the curriculum for teaching health skills is not much different than other curricular areas. It can be done by a classroom teacher for his or her group of children, or a group of teachers may get together to develop a sequential plan for each grade level. For health education curriculum planning, it is essential that educators and health professionals work together. The following steps can be used in curriculum planning.

Step 1: Assessment of Needs and Resources

Each community is different in the health needs of its children. Though an elaborate needs assessment is helpful, it is not an actuality possible for most communities. Teachers can meet with parents and health care providers, however, to determine their perceptions of children's health needs at the various developmental levels. Available data or short questionnaires can be used to determine children's experiences with illness or the major health problems characteristic of the particular group of children. In addition, it would be helpful to obtain some direct assessment of the children's current patterns of health behavior.

Assessment of resources includes both school and community. What teaching activities and materials are already in the curriculum that might be related to general areas of health skills? Are there some health professionals or parents who would be willing to assist with a health education program?

Step 2: Curriculum Development

Form a curriculum development group to include: teachers, school nurse, physician, parents, and other health professionals (dentist, psychologist, nutritionist, and so on). This group could start by reviewing literature and curricula from other sources. Based on the review plus the needs assessment, the group should state the program goals in terms of general skills to be developed by the children. Next, state specific health skills to be developed within each general skill area. Review and evaluate available teaching methodologies, teaching aids, and student materials related to the specific health skills. Finally, design learning activities (content and process) to help children develop the health skills, and plan for opportunities for practice.

Step 3: Teacher Preparation

Identify teacher competencies necessary for carrying out the health education activities. If new content and process are to be used in the activities, locate individuals who can provide in-service training. If in-service training is needed, conduct the training and evaluate its effectiveness in terms of developing the necessary competence.

Step 4: Implementation and Evaluation

Schedule the sequence of learning activities for the teaching of health skills. Collect any preprogram data that will be used as part of the evaluation. As the program is conducted, a means should be provided for monitoring students' progress in the development of skills. To support and reinforce learning, attempt to provide parent education activities to correspond with classroom learning activities. It is also important to coordinate activities with health services and pupil services to provide additional resources for children needing individualized attention. At the end of the period of instruction, data should be collected to determine as much as possible the extent to which children did develop the stated health skills.

Health Education for Target Groups

In all schools there will be certain groups of children, such as asthmatic children, who have specific health problems and special educational needs that cannot be met through the health education curriculum. Once a means of identifying these children can be established, they can constitute a target group for which the school health program can develop special education activities. A few examples of possible target groups include: pregnant teen-agers, children with seizure disorders, students who want to quit smoking, children severely deficient in interpersonal skills, and students with problems related to drug or alcohol abuse. Health professionals have the awareness and knowledge of major health problems of children within a community. They can assist schools in identifying appropriate target groups of children that can benefit from specific health education programs. Such a process might include screening programs to identify children with particular problems or working with community physicians to bring together parents and children that have particular health problems. Physicians are more likely to have ongoing contacts with parents and are in a position to encourage parents to participate in health education programs. The physician can also assist in interpreting the objectives and values of health education programs for particular target groups.

School health education programs can offer the opportunity of reaching larger numbers of children with particular health problems. In primary care settings, it may be difficult to devote sufficient time for doing health education on a one-to-one basis. By bringing children and their families together, however, it might be possible to utilize blocks of time to meet the health education needs for a larger number of children and their families. Working as a team, educational personnel and health professionals can meet with children and parents to deal with the particular health concerns of a special target group. For example, it would be very difficult on a one-to-one basis to devote sufficient time to help adolescents deal with the implications of teen-age pregnancy. By meeting with pregnant teen-agers as a group, however, it might be possible to help them deal more effectively with the experience they are going through as well as to assist them in developing the parenting skills and child health care skills that they will need.

Health education programs for target groups should result in outcomes that will improve the health of the children or improve the ability of the families to cope with a particular health problem. The health care providers who see the children or the families as part of their routine health care are in a position to evaluate the effectiveness of such programs. Are the children improving in health status? Are the families coping more effectively with a particular health problem? Teachers see the children function within the context of daily activities and can make direct observation of coping and improved abilities. Thus, the concept of educational and health professionals working together is further emphasized in the evaluation of health education programs.

Challenge

Unlike illness care, which intervenes at particular defined occurrences of ill health, preventive medicine and health maintenance is an ongoing, lifetime process. It must begin at a very young age and be carried on through adulthood to develop competencies that will enable people to assume greater responsibility for their own health. As far as children are concerned, the one thing that most have in common is that they participate in and attend schools. It is obvious that if there is to be an impact on the quality of life through improved health behavior, the school health program offers one critical interface for health care providers, educators, and families to work together to meet the health needs of the children.

REFERENCES

1. I. Illich, *Deschooling Society* (New York: Harper & Row, 1972), p. 1.

2. K. J. Connolly and J. S. Bruner, "Competence: Its Nature and Nurture," in Connolly and Bruner, Eds., *The Growth of Competence* (New York: Academic Press, 1973), p. 3.

3. *Preventive Medici.le, USA: Health Promotion and Consumer Health Education.* A Task Force Report sponsored by the John E. Fogarty International Center for Advanced Study in the Health Sciences, National Institutes of Health and the American College of Preventive Medicine, Part I, Life Style and Health Status (New York: Prodist, 1976), p. 6.

4. E. Newberger, C. M. Newberger, and J. B. Richmond, "Child Health in America: Toward a Rational Public Policy," *Milbank Memorial Fund Quarterly* 54, no. 3 (Summer 1976): 249.

5. *Ibid.*

6. H. Knobloch and B. Pasamanich, "Prospective Studies in the Epidemiology of Reproductive Causality: Methods, Findings and Some Implications," *Merrill-Palmer Quarterly of Behavior and Development* 12, no. 1 (1966): 27.

7. P. M. Fitzhardinge and E. M. Stevens, "The Small for Date Infant, II: Neurological and Intellectual Sequelae," *Pediatrics* 50, no. 1 (July 1972): 50.

8. J. B. Henshaw, A. P. Scheiner, A. W. Moxly, L. Gaer, and V. Abel, "School Failure and Deafness after Silent Congenital Cytomegalovirus Infection," *New England Journal of Medicine* 295, no. 9 (August 26, 1976): 468.

9. P. S. Klein, G. B. Forbes, and P. R. Nader, "Effects of Starvation in Infancy (Pyloric Stenosis) on Subsequent Learning Abilities," *Journal of Pediatrics* 87, no. 1 (July 1975): 8.

10. Newberger *et al., op. cit.*

11. *Ibid.*

12. *Ibid.*

13. R. J. Haggerty, K. Roghmann, and I. B. Pless, Eds., *Child Health and the Community* (New York: John Wiley and Sons, 1975).

14. J. M. Krager and D. J. Safer, "Type and Prevalence of Medication Used in the Treatment of Hyperactive Children," *New England Journal of Medicine* 291, no. 21 (Nov. 21, 1974): 1118.

15. *Preventive Medicine, USA, op. cit.*

16. *Ibid.*

17. E. M. Sliepcevich, *School Health Education Study: A Summary Report* (Washington, D.C.: School Health Education Study, 1964).

18. *Health Education: A Conceptual Approach to Curriculum Design* (Washington, D.C.: School Health Education Study, 1967).

19. U.S. Department of Health, Education, and Welfare, *The Report of the President's Committee on Health Education* (Washington, D.C.: U.S. Government Printing Office, 1973), p. 21.

20. *Ibid.*

21. L. W. Green, *Determining the Impact and Effectiveness of Health Education as It Relates to Federal Policy* (Washington, D.C.: U.S. Department of Health, Education and Welfare, Office of the Deputy Assistant Secretary for Planning and Evaluation, 1976).

22. *Ibid.,* p. 9.

23. *Ibid.*

24. *Ibid.*

25. J. Elliott and K. J. Connolly, "Hierarchical Structure in Skill Development," in Connolly and Bruner *op. cit.*, p. 135.

26. Connolly and Bruner, *op. cit.*, p. 5.

27. C.E. Lewis and M.A. Lewis, "Child-Initiated Care," A study of the determinants of the illness behavior of children. U.S. Dept. of Commerce; National Technical Information Service No. 253726, prepared for National Center for Health Services Research; 1974.

28. J. D. Swisher, "Mental Health—The Core of Preventive Health Education," *Journal of School Health* 46, no. 7 (Sept. 1976): 386-391.

29. *Life Skills for Health: Focus on Mental Health* (Raleigh, N.C.: Division of Health, Safety, and Physical Education, North Carolina Department of Public Instruction, 1974).

Chapter 2

Health and Education: Linked for the Child and Family

A Model for Planning of School Health Programs

Philip R. Nader, M.D.

It seems obvious to state that school health programs are affected by the families they serve, by the schoolteachers and administrators with whom they interact daily, and by the providers of general and specialty health care in the community. Yet, when school health fails to live up to its potential, it usually means that inadequate attention has been paid to how these three systems interact to influence a specific desired outcome. For example, a child is found on vision screening to be in need of referral for glasses. Yet, six months later the child does not have glasses and is failing reading. What routine follow-up activities should have been brought into play to prevent this failure? What was known about the family and the resources ahead of time to match the details of the screening program to the nature of the local community?

HOME AND FAMILY

Each facet of the system (home, school, health care providers) has different perceptions, priorities, and values; any of these differences can be a barrier. Such barriers frequently keep the systems from complementing each other in working toward the benefit of the child's health and educational well-being. School health is the natural arena where these three systems come together. This chapter will examine each system's particular perceptions of health, priorities in health, and values for health, which need to be thought about in planning new programs or changing existing ones.

Children are, for the most part, passive recipients of health care. Both the home and school place this constraint of passivity on children. Health care providers often reinforce this passive role and rely on mothers to initiate and maintain health care. This is dramatically illustrated by observing the lack of direct verbal communication with children during visits for health services.[1]

School health programs should help the children become active participants and decision makers regarding their own health care.[2] This will have to be done by giving children the opportunity to practice decision-making skills regarding their health at school and by working with parents to reinforce the child's role. Naturally, the ability of the children to make decisions about health care depends on their age and cognitive development, their concepts of health and illness,[3] and the social learning that has taken place in the family.[4] The ability of parents to allow children to participate to the degree that they can in decision making about health is dependent on how they themselves were reared and their comfort with the parental role of guide rather than of dictator.

One way the school could help children learn about the appropriate use of health services is to institute a decision-making model of interaction wth pupils as they come to the health office for minor complaints.[5] For example, the inquiry technique of "what do you think you should do about your skinned knee?" replaces "come here while I wash off your skinned knee." Various alternatives that the child comes up with are explored with him, along with the possible consequences of various actions the child chooses or does not choose. Final decision making is not relinquished to the child if that decision would be harmful or unhealthy. But by exploring a child's feelings when he or she visits the nurse for headaches or stomachaches, school health personnel will find that child increasingly able to identify the "real" sources of stress that are resulting in a somatic complaint (for example, a "math headache").

This approach can be expanded to allow children to make the original decision to visit the school health office by removing the requirement to obtain permission to go to the nurse, which constrains children to remain passive in their health care. Schools that use this system find that no more than the usual number of students utilize the health services. In one study of visits to the elementary school nurse in a "campus" school setting where permission to go to the nurse was not required, most children who did go discussed the idea of going to the nurse with a friend or teacher before the visit.[6] This would indicate that children also might go through a "validation of sick role behavior" much as adults do.

In interaction with parents about children's visits or complaints discussed with the nurse, the child's role in participating in decision making can be reinforced. Parents usually respond positively to the idea that by giving children certain responsibilities they gain maturity and self-confidence. Overly anxious parents will need support from the health professional. What are the sources of anxiety? Is the mother overly worried about minor illness in the child because of a fear that the child is "sickly" and "almost died as an infant," or does she have incomplete knowledge about the nature of a chronic illness such as asthma or epilepsy?

D. Mechanic studied the health and illness behaviors of 350 mother-child pairs (with selection of the children from the fourth and eighth grades).[7] Although the overall results indicate little maternal influence in determining children's patterns of illness behavior, it was found that family stress made mothers more likely to report symptoms for themselves and for their children. They were also more likely to contact the doctor concerning their children's health.

A school health program could respond quickly to evidence of children's and families' stess. The works of R. J. Haggerty, K. Roghmann, and others [8,9,10] have documented the impact of family stress and coping patterns on the use of health services (telephone and emergency room visits). Frequent visits to the nurse can signal stress in either the home or school environment of the child. Home visits or contacts should be made on all frequent visitors to the health office. Often the ability of a family to marshall the resources to deal effectively with a health problem in the child relates to the pattern established for dealing with acute stress events superimposed on more chronic stress, such as poverty, unemployment, chronic illness in adult family members, or marital disagreements. Sometimes the inability to handle a child's health problem is merely a result of not having the practice of getting through the "systems" of health care, of not knowing the procedures for obtaining appointments, or of not having experienced the value of being involved in planning for the child's care. Appropriate outreach activities by health service allied professionals can aid immensely in working with such families to increase their knowledge of community resources, to increase a sense of trust in the school personnel, and to foster independence in assuming responsibility for dealing with their child's health problems. Over an extended period, it might, in fact, be possible to alter the coping styles and strengths that families have available to deal with stress when it inevitably appears.

THE SCHOOL

It has been stated, perhaps unfairly, that schools are for adults and not children; yet few would argue that adult attitudes and expectations influence the school's role in dealing with health problems and health promotion. Both parent-child and teacher-child interactions are based on knowledge, beliefs, and experiences that often do not allow them to respond most effectively to children. School personnel often have insufficient knowledge of child development or health needs. Previous experiences with health care providers may cause inappropriate fear, lack of understanding, or unrealistic expectations of "magical intervention" by the health professional.

Common examples include concern on the part of teachers about showing moving pictures to epileptic students for fear of precipitating a seizure, ascribing chewing on pencils and other forms of pica to mineral or other dietary deficiencies, and excessive attention to children subject to attacks of "asthma." Other unrealistic expectations commonly encountered include the value of a "brain wave" or "medication" in helping a behavioral and educational problem child.

School health programs have an obligation to attempt to overcome these knowledge and attitudinal barriers through education. Teachers are generally enthusiastically receptive to joint efforts at in-service training on some of these health-related areas, if administrators can be convinced of their value over more "pressing" educational priorities. The support of concerned community parents can be essential in establishing a priority for such teacher seminars. These parents may also be valuable in securing health care professionals from the community to be resources for such seminars. Health care providers will gain insight into the problems faced by educators through mutual participation in health-related seminars.

Health education and promotion of health often have low priorities in the curriculum. Seminars such as the ones described above can stimulate interest. Another avenue might be to develop health education programs outside the formal curriculum that are specifically focused on children with specialized educational needs or those with consequences of a health or developmental problem. Examples include children with physical handicaps or chronic illnesses. Outcomes should be predicted and measured: improved educational performance, better social adjustment, and improved school attendance for the child; and better understanding of the nature of the problem and improved coping skills for the child, his parents, and his teachers.

THE HEALTH CARE SYSTEM

For today's school-age children and adolescents, the "new morbidity" and major unmet health needs are dental, emotional, and learning problems, making decisions about sexual behavior, problems associated with alcohol and drug use, and coping with chronic handicapping conditions. These clearly stand out as striking, even in areas where more "traditional" health problems are prevalent.[11-14] It becomes necessary, therefore, to develop school health programs and activities with these "health problem" needs in mind.

Health care providers (as well as parents and teachers), however, are handicapped by their lack of knowledge and experience in dealing with these health concerns. Difficulties may also result from working in an environment that traditionally has emphasized disease and episodic illness care more often than health maintenance, comprehensive primary health, or preventive medicine. Such orientation and training often leave health care providers ill equipped to learn firsthand the numerous physical health and mental health problems that are undetected and untreated in a community. This environment also inhibits the development of health care providers' roles in prevention and early detection of these problems.

It has been suggested that a modification of G. Caplan's preventive health model[15] be adapted by primary health care providers working collaboratively with school systems. Primary preventive activities are those that improve the school environment. Secondary preventive activities are those that relate to early detection of conditions inimical to a child's sound physical, social, or educational growth. Tertiary preventive activities are case/patient/family-oriented. They aim to rehabilitate existing problems and reach the optimal level of function for a given handicapping condition. Examples are illustrated in Table 2-1.

For example, a practicing pediatrician in a group practice caring for the majority of students in schools of a given geographic area is retained by that district as a school medical consultant for one day per week. In the area of primary prevention, a portion of the physician's time is spent in in-service sessions with teachers on developmental variations normally observed in young elementary school children. This service improves the general milieu of the school environment, and the teacher's self-confidence is reinforced in observing normal variation without unnecessary labeling of children as "deviant" or "problematic." This interaction also benefits the physician who desires an opportunity to practice preventive medicine and sees this consultation route as a potential avenue to influencing a large number of children, compared with the relatively minute number of children on whom he could have an impact in the one-to-one office setting.

In secondary and tertiary areas, the health care provider has his horizons widened by teaming with school personnel in the evaluation

Table 2-1 Preventive School Health Care

Type	Definition	Examples
Primary	Improves school milieu, or supports school environment of all children, or identifies special high-risk groups	Program to define and help children failing in school
		Program helping teachers learn more about normal variability in child development
		Teen pregnancy program incorporating parenting skills
Secondary	Early identification of problems likely to interfere with school or healthy functioning	Learning disability screening that includes programs of remedies and recognizes potential hazards of labeling
		Scoliosis screening program
Tertiary	Returns identified health problem to as normal a state as possible	Case conferences and problem-solving activities for children and families with numerous conditions such as chronic handicapping conditions (arthritis, diabetes, seizures, allergies, asthma, obesity, physically deforming conditions, learning problems, and school phobia)

Source: Reproduced with permission from P.R. Nader, "The School Health Service: Making Primary Care Effective," *Pediatric Clinics of North America* 21, no. 1 (Feb. 1974): 57.

and management of pupils who have learning or adjustment problems. He could find out important information related to the future development of his patients that might not otherwise have been brought to his attention by parents. School personnel, through this kind of interaction, will also benefit by not feeling isolated in attempting to deal with the problems and by having support from a professional who is highly respected by parents. In all areas, the family and child should benefit from the increased communication that would naturally occur among concerned professionals.

Adequate access to health care also requires joint efforts between the home, the source of care, and the school. When the health care systems are not utilized, providers often may blame poor family attitudes or lack of motivation or knowledge, without paying enough attention to issues of trust, confidence, and the processes of priorities and decision making that everyone must go through before participating in curative or preventive health services.

The school health service offers an obvious setting to assist in this process of providing smooth and adequate access to health care.[16] A school health program has the opportunity for interaction with the child in the role of "student" rather than "patient." This is especially attractive to many who view school health as a possible vehicle for overcoming some of the actual or perceived barriers that block adequate access to a health care system. This will necessitate going beyond the usual home visit following a written notification to a parent of a child's health problem.[17] It may even entail in some instances placing direct services (for example, a dental clinic) in the school. Access can be enhanced by providing school health nurses with more skills in problem assessment and management (such as school nurse practitioners).[18-21] It will also include providing outreach workers who can become familiar with both families and services, as well as developing more formal relationships between individual schools and specific sources of health care for children. Finally, more physicians must be adequately trained to handle school health consultative services.[22-24]

REFERENCES

1. D. MacCarthy, "Communication Between Children and Doctors," *Development Medicine and Child Neurology* 16, no. 3 (Feb. 1974): 279.

2. G. Parcel, "Skills Approach to Health Education: A Framework for Integrating Cognitive and Affective Learning," *Journal of School Health* 46, no. 7 (Sept. 1976): 403.

3. D. S. Gochman, "Children's Perceptions of Vulnerability to Illness and Accidents," *Health Services and Mental Health Administration Health Reports* 86 (March 1971): 247.

4. Carter L. Marshall, K. M. Hassanein, R. S. Hassanein, and C. L. Paul, "Attitudes Toward Health Among Children of Different Races and Socioeconomic Status," *Pediatrics* 46, no. 3 (Sept. 1970): 422.

5. B. Palmer and C. E. Lewis, "Development of Health Attitudes and Behaviors," *Journal of School Health* 46, no. 7 (Sept. 1976): 401.

6. W. Van Arsdale, K. Roghmann, and P. Nader, "Visits to an Elementary School Nurse," *Journal of School Health* 42, no. 3 (March 1972): 142.

7. D. Mechanic, "The Influences of Mothers on their Children's Health Attitude and Behavior," *Pediatrics* 33, no. 3 (March 1966): 444.

8. R. J. Meyer and R. J. Haggerty, "Streptococcal Infections in Families: Factors Altering Susceptibility," *Pediatrics* 29, no. 4 (April 1962): 539.

9. K. Roghmann and R. J. Haggerty, "Family Stress and the Use of Health Services," *International Journal of Epidemiology* 1, no. 3 (Sept. 1972): 279.

10. K. Roghmann and R. J. Haggerty, "The Stress Model for Illness Behavior," in Haggerty, Roghmann, and I.B. Pless, Eds., *Child Health and the Community* (New York: John Wiley and Sons, 1975), pp. 142-156.

11. I.B. Pless and B. Satterwhite, "Chronic Illness," in Haggerty *et al., op. cit.*, pp. 78-94.

12. P.R. Nader, "The Frequency and Nature of School Problems: The New Morbidity," in Hagerty *et al, op. cit.*, pp. 101-105.

13. P. R. Nader, A. Emmel, and E. Charney, "The School Health Service: A New Model," *Pediatrics* 49, no. 5 (May 1972): 805.

14. K. Hein, M. Cohen, and I. Litt, "Planning Health Services for Urban Adolescents," *Urban Health* 4, no. 1 (Feb. 1975): 28.

15. G. Caplan, *Principles of Preventive Psychiatry* (New York: Basic Books, 1964).

16. L. A. Aday and R. Anderson, *Development of Indices of Access to Medical Care* (Ann Arbor: Health Administration Press, 1975).

17. J.G. Caufman, E.A. Warburton, and C.S. Shultz, "Health Care of School Children: Effective Referral Patterns," *American Journal of Public Health* 59, no. 1 (Jan. 1969): 86.

18. J. M. Bellaire, "School Nurse Practitioner Program," *American Journal of Nursing* 71, no. 11 (Nov. 1971): 2192.

19. H. K. Silver, "The School Nurse Practitioner Program: A New and Expanded Role for the School Nurse," *Journal of American Medical Association* 216, no. 8 (May 1971): 1332.

20. J. Conrad, "The High School Nurse as a Pediatric Nurse Practitioner," *Pediatric Nursing* no. 6 (Nov./Dec. 1975): 15-17.

21. C.E. Lewis, A. Lorimer, B. Lindeman, B. Palmer, and M.A. Lewis, "An Evaluation of the Impact of School Nurse Practitioners," *Journal of School Health* 44, no. 6 (June 1974): 331.

22. M. G. Wagner, L. S. Levin, and M. H. Heller, "The School Physician, a Study of Satisfaction with His Role," *Pediatrics* 40, no. 6 (Dec. 1967): 1009.

23. M. J. Senn, "The Role, Prerequisites and Training of the School Physician," *Pediatric Clinics of North America* 12, no. 4 (Nov. 1965): 1039.

24. M. Kappelman, P. Roberts, R. Rinaldi, and M. Cornblath, "The School Health Team and the School Physician," *American Journal of Diseases of Children* 129, no. 2 (Feb. 1975): 191.

Chapter 3

School Health vs. Health in the School: Integrating Medical and Educational Models

Katherine P. Messenger, M.C.P.,
Philip R. Nader, M.D.,
Guy S. Parcel, Ph.D.,
Philip J. Porter, M.D., and
Mildred C. Williamson, R.N.

Putting school health together means putting together different institutions and agencies such as schools, school boards, health centers, hospitals, and public health departments. It also means putting people together who have different training and skills, such as nurses, doctors, teachers, guidance counselors, aides, special education experts, and others. This often results in a complex set of administrative, programmatic, and interpersonal interactions that strongly influence attempts to develop or change school health programs.

This chapter will first consider an oft-neglected element—the different conceptual frameworks within which both institutions and personnel work. By considering a generalized and somewhat polarized model of each institution's framework, the reader will then appreciate the basis for the differing sets of assumptions and values that guide the respective professionals' practice and image. It should become clear why barriers exist to the development of optimal school health programs.

THEORETICAL FRAMEWORKS

We will then give examples of two successful, innovative school health program models—one set basically in the health system and the other primarily in the educational system. How these programs developed will be described, as well as the nature of the activities. Emphasis will be placed on identification of common barriers that program developers ran into in melding these two rather distinct professional worlds.

The different theoretical frameworks of educators and health professionals include their definition of their profession (what does it mean to say that one is a doctor or a teacher?), the nature of their everyday work and interpersonal relationships (what is the difference between the doctor/patient and teacher/student interaction?), and their expectations of outcome (what are the goals of medicine and education?). The conceptual frameworks under which the two professions operate can be characterized in four broad categories: conditions of work, orientation of work, professional attributes, and constraints on work.

Conditions of Work

Where do doctors and teachers work, and what are the important attributes of those settings that might differentiate them?

The work of medicine occurs in a variety of settings, from doctors' offices to clinics to emergency rooms to intensive care units. These settings are often unfamiliar to the patient and awesome or frightening in their equipment, bustling activity, and general ambience. Most people visit them rarely or episodically, usually for specific purposes, with immediate needs, or even with fear. The patients whom the doctor sees have come voluntarily or at his specific request. The immediate context of any situation in which medical work is performed usually involves an individual patient and clinician. Other clinicians or allied health personnel may be present for parts of the encounter, and parents of children are usually the only others present. Encounters are time-limited.

Teaching work on the other hand occurs in standardized settings—classrooms in school buildings. Groups of children, who are required to be there, are the responsibility of one teacher (or, occasionally, a team of teachers with an aide or two). Encounters last for periods of one hour (in secondary school) to hours at a time (in primary grades), five days a week, nine months a year, for up to 12 years. Although the overall patterns within the setting (class periods, gym, recess, and so on) are well understood, their daily manifestations are more nearly random—or at least unpredictable.

> In the small but crowded world of the classroom, events come and go with astonishing rapidity. There is evidence, as we have seen, to show that the elementary school teacher typically engages in 200 or 300 interpersonal interchanges every hour of her working day. Moreover, although that number may remain fairly stable from hour to hour, the content and sequence of those interchanges cannot be predicted or preplanned with any

exactitude. In short, classrooms are not neat and orderly places even though some educational theories make them sound as if they are or should be. This does not mean that there is no order in educational affairs (indeed, some teachers strive so hard to maintain some semblance of order that they lose sight of everything else), but the structure underlying these kaleidoscopic events is not easily discerned, nor is it, except superficially, under the control of the teacher.[1]

The only medical setting that approaches this fast-paced and uncontrollable stream of events is the busy emergency room. Yet, the surface variation in classroom life reduces to a relatively small range of types of variation: disruptive students, administrative intrusions, field trips, "bad days," serendipitous teaching opportunity, and so on. Each requires a response of flexibility, rapid recovery, or iron control. In the delivery of medicine, however, the surface quality of everyday work changes less, but the types of work vary more and the responses required are different: each patient is seen as unique, and diagnostic peculiarities and individual effects of treatment often require specific responses: consultations, searches of the literature, referrals, and so on.

Whether one perceives a new setting as suitable for effective work depends in part on how much it resembles settings where that person was trained or worked previously. Because medical and educational settings are so different, combining their work in the processes of more effective school health will require careful planning and, probably, greater overlap during training.

Orientation of Work

What does it mean to *do* medicine, to *do* teaching? What is the behavior that is most often considered appropriate, behavior that D. C. Lortie[2] has termed "preoccupations, beliefs and preferences?"

Pathology vs. Normality

Probably the single most important difference is that medical work is oriented toward *pathology*, whereas teaching is oriented toward *normality*. Seeing the doctor is something we do when we are sick, when we suspect we might be sick, or when we want to prevent illness. Going to school in this country is something done by *almost* everyone of certain ages.[3] Learning is something that, to some extent, occurs naturally as part of growing up and becoming an adult. Schools and teaching exist to foster learning, to standardize its occurrence, and to direct its course (socialization). In the doctor's office, the well person is out of place, a user of efforts better devoted to those who "need care." In the classroom, the pathologic is disruptive of regular procedures.

Individual vs. Groups

Medical work is focused heavily on the individual and results in a case management approach to service. Educational work is concentrated on reaching groups of children simultaneously. This group orientation and allegiance is more ambivalent and frustrating than the medical model, because in American education the ideal is to allow each child to achieve to the best of his or her ability. This might require special attention or individualized approaches. Indeed, many of the personal rewards of teaching come from evidences of individual performance, pleasure, or learning. But "... the ideals of American public schools include two principles: the importance of equity in treatment and the assumption that all children can benefit from schooling. The structure makes it difficult (although not impossible) to openly favor particular children or to argue that some children cannot be taught."[4]

The principles underlying medical work are not the same. Although an ethical commitment to treat all in need prevails, there is no assumption that everyone can benefit from medical care or that it is a *right* (although this concept is gaining support). More emphasis is placed on "do no harm" and quality standards of care than on universality and uniformity. In addition, deviations from a standard of equity are far less obvious and, thus, less troubling to the physician because of the individual, private nature of interactions.

Treatment vs. Interaction

Physicians, in large part, diagnose and prescribe or treat. To do this work, specific tools and procedures—often forbidden to anyone other than doctors—are employed. Although caring, relieving anxiety, and counseling are part of medical work, they are not, in practice, its core.

> The physician sees himself as a professionally competent person who is in a social position to apply scientific knowledge and to exercise impartial control over the situation in order to achieve the rational goal of curing or helping a sick patient. The patient's part of the job is to trust the doctor and cooperate with him.[5]

In many cases, however, the doctor (or nurse) can achieve results without the patient's active participation. As long as the patient provides his bodily presence, the operation can be successful, the shots can be given, the bone set.

Teaching, on the other hand, is intensely interactional work. Teachers cannot *make* children learn without some degree of cooperation and shared goals. To be effective, they cannot rely on special tools and enforced treatment but must work more pragmatically and opportunistically with children to involve them in the learning process. They thus have a much greater appreciation than does the clinician "of how the immediate social setting gives shape and meaning to human behavior."[6]

P. W. Jackson, on the basis of his observations and interviews, has characterized the good classroom in terms of *immediacy, informality, autonomy,* and *individuality.* Although autonomy would probably occur in physicians' or health workers' characterizations of the good office or clinic, the other three would not. More likely to be included would be the characteristics of the resources: *completeness, order, cleanliness,* and *professionalism.*

It is interesting to note that the areas in which the medical treatment model fails are those in which the patient has to be part of the process, when he or she has to learn a modified life style or confront psychological problems. These are the strengths of the interactional education model. Until the models are merged in practice, a misfit continues to occur.

Life vs. Knowledge

Finally, one more, perhaps obvious, distinction in orientation can be drawn. Behind the often trivial and ordinary activities of much medical care lies the awareness on the part of both doctor and patient that the relationship could be a matter of life or death. A routine immunization could be preventing a deadly disease; a headache and fever might be meningitis.

Educational work has little of this aura, which lends suspense, prestige, and awesomeness to medical work. The positive reward lies in a life enriched with knowledge—any life or death threat is low-keyed: without a good education, one may be doomed to a poor and unrewarding life. The rewards, however, are far off and uncertain; few children or teachers believe that message completely. Thus, motivating and engaging students in the educational process or sustaining teachers' faith in the importance of what they are doing depends more on individual circumstances in education. The everyday routine, inconvenience, and unpleasantness of medical work are sustained and made significant by the specter of the medical emergency and the miracle cure. The everyday routine of teaching must rest much more on its own merits.

The portion of medical work that is most relevant to school health, however— ambulatory and well-child care— is least amenable to the "life or death" posture. As in education, the process is mundane, the potential rewards are in the future, and the threats are not apparent. With the control of infectious childhood diseases and the improvement of living standards, few children die or become seriously ill. The influence of the medical life and death model has been reduced.

Professional Attributes

The most basic difference in professional attributes between teachers and physicians is the relative insecurity or partiality of teaching as a profession compared with medicine. Medicine is the most fully developed profession, through its extensive command of scientific knowledge, esoteric skills and procedures, its monopoly over setting the conditions of work and of entry into the profession, and its prestigious status.[7] These factors lead to self-assurance about one's position and the value of one's work. They also lead to the assumption and—to keep up the image of the profession—the demand that one be a leader and not be directed in one's work by others. By being a full profession, medicine has been protected from public or lay scrutiny and oversight.

Education is another matter. As Lortie points out, teaching is only incompletely a profession.[8] Entry remains easy; training is varied, less scientifically and intellectually rigorous, and less sustained.

Being a teacher (as opposed to being a professor) sets one apart only slightly from other occupations. Still, teaching has traditionally been a highly regarded (and at times almost sacred) calling, and its preeminence is tied to its crucial role in preparing the young to be members of the society. Conditions of work, entry into the profession, and oversight are in the control of laymen: principals, administrators, school boards, voters. Teaching is a "partial profession" with a "special, but shadowed" status.[9] One of the results of this situation is that teachers can have much greater ambivalence about the true nature of their work (are they employees or professionals?) and less self-assurance about the respect and status due them. Thus, they are likely to resent intrusions into their work or space and to be defensive about the value of their own methods.

The other health professions— nursing, for example— have much in common with teaching. They are subordinate to medical authority in most situations, the change in their status with training and licensure is less sharp, they are ambivalent about their professionalism and status, and they have been unable to define fully autonomous models.

Science vs. Common Sense,
Technology vs. Human Ingenuity

A second difference in professional orientation is the mode of thought and work imparted or emphasized in training and practice. Jackson characterizes practicing teachers by the nontechnical vocabulary and conceptual simplicity of their talk.[10]

Although doctors often engage in extremely simplistic talk and explanations to patients, their talk among themselves and their style of work are generally highly technical, scientific, and rational in approach. General practitioners may exhibit a closed-mindedness (or belief in their tried and true ways of doing things) and an intuitive approach, but in much of medical work there is a strong emphasis on keeping up with the latest advances, maintaining a scientific approach to problem solving, the systematic codification of experience, and indeed a fascination with new procedures. Certainly, medical training (and other health training) places a distinctly different emphasis on science, rational problem solving, and research from that of teacher training. Medical training is also more systematically and intensively clinical; doctors learn by doing under critical eyes for many years. Martin Meyer has commented caustically, "Medical training would be more like teacher training if two-thirds of the time were devoted to rephrasing and discussing the Hippocratic Oath."[11] It is interesting to note, however, that beneath the surface complexity of "scientific" medicine is a relatively simple underlying view of causality: organisms or other external agents invade the body and create dysfunction.

But we all have far greater firsthand experience with teaching, teachers, and schools than we have with microbiology, healing, and doctors. Although medical work might, in fact, be no more of a science than teaching and its effect on health no more predictable or substantial, our limited exposure to it maintains the mystery. Classrooms are too familiar to be awesome. The variations we have seen between good and bad teachers and classroom techniques, along with the lack of substantial "breakthroughs" (most classrooms look and feel very much like the ones we attended as children) reduce the public's awe of teaching and increase the feeling that "anyone can do it."

This attitude of familiarity affects the training process also. Prospective teachers are more likely to have strong preexisting views on teaching work and can be less powerfully resocialized through preprofessional education than medical students. In addition, teacher education has virtually none of the "rites of passage" intensity of clinical medical education.[12]

Constraints on Work

Three types of constraints on success and satisfaction differentiate medical from educational work: ineffective intervention, lack of cooperation, and institutional barriers.

Ineffective Intervention

Medical work is most often limited by a general lack of understanding of certain disease processes and their effective therapy—many cancers fall into this category. It is limited periodically by the unavailability of known therapies or services (for example, not enough kidney dialysis machines or no emergency medical services in a remote area) and by doctor inattention or error. In all but the last instance, the individual physician (or other health worker) need feel little *personal* ineffectiveness or personal helplessness.

Teaching, on the other hand, might be ineffective at times because of systematic or distributional gaps in knowledge and services (for example, a shortage of bilingual teachers or special supplies for the blind or deaf), but in most cases it fails for unknown reasons. Because of the intensely interpersonal and idiosyncratic nature of classroom teaching, teachers are more likely to feel personally at fault when a child is not reached or they are more likely not to know *where* to place the blame. (Did they not try the right approaches? Will the child show the results later? Has some earlier teacher done the damage?) In other words, teaching is more likely to cause internalized feelings of ineffectiveness. Doctors turn failure into demands for more research, more hospitals, and so on; teachers are more likely to retreat further into their classrooms.

Lack of Cooperation

Physicians and teachers share one powerful constraint: the uncooperative patient, the inattentive student, and troublesome parents. In this situation, the orientation of teaching work offers greater support. When the nature of work is seen as interpersonal and contextual and when one knows some students are not there by choice, one can accept a degree of incongruence between teaching goals and pupil or parent ones. In fact, a certain percentage of uninterested students free the teacher's time to focus on the most receptive and interesting group members; only disruptive behavior causes real problems.

Doctors, on the other hand, tend to be more condemning of all who do not follow their instructions, question their judgments, or appear disinterested in their efforts. Perhaps because of the doctors' higher professional status and the deference to which they are accustomed, the experience is more unsettling than to teachers who are more realistic or modest about expected respect and results.

Support can also be lacking from colleagues. In general, physicians can demand support from other health workers, nurses, social workers, technicians, and so on. Lack of support is often synonymous with insubordination. Interphysician problems usually reflect status and power differences within the profession (family practitioners who "lose" patients to medical center specialists, and so on). Teachers, on the other hand, have few people under their direction. Lack of support is usually manifested by not being backed up by principals and administrators or being undercut by them.

Institutional Barriers

"At the basis of teacher status is the indisputable constraint that without access to a position in the schools the teacher cannot practice his craft."[13] The license to practice medicine does not require institutional support, approval, or setting to be used. Although many physicians do work in or for institutions, their options are greater than those of teachers. Other health personnel are more like teachers in terms of constraints on their practice settings. Furthermore, the vast majority of school settings are public, whereas most medical settings (even institutional ones such as hospitals) are private. Any institution imposes certain constraints on the individual: red tape, rules, bureaucratic procedures, and lack of freedom in practice and innovation. Public institutions, especially those as visible and integral to local politics as are schools, add further constraints through lay control, oversight, budgeting hassles, and more bureaucratic red tape. The conditions and style of work oblige greater compromise with professional and individual goals and preferences.

INTEGRATING THE MEDICAL AND EDUCATIONAL FRAMEWORKS

We have found substantial discrepancies between the medical and the educational frameworks, variations along a number of scales: pathology/normality, individual/group, scientific empiricism/eclectic pragmatism, professional dominance/"shadowed status," and unequal control over the choice of settings for and conditions of work. Contemplation of these theoretical frameworks can be frustrating or annoying; they may seem stereotypic or unreal, unrelated to everyday problems of establishing or refashioning a school health program. We can make the transition to the real world, however, by considering more carefully the range of actual practice and values in both the educational and health worlds.

Some doctors and health personnel think and talk as teachers, and vice versa. Some teachers are more interested in cognitive learning styles, behavior modification techniques, Piagetian theory, or evaluation than others. Some physicians are becoming more interested and better trained in psychosocial medicine, child development, doctor-patient interactions, group techniques, and health education. One can perceive trends toward greater individualized learning plans within public schools, greater attention to diagnostic tests, and a wider variety of learning settings and techniques. Within the health care field, professional dominance and private settings are partially giving way to community health planning, team approaches, public oversight, and more standardized and universal care settings. Health workers and reading specialists who combine an individual diagnosis and disease orientation with group interventions and educational programs are growing in number.

From this perspective, the prospects for creative school health programs would appear great, though there are "deviant" values and iconoclastic individuals within each model to be more systematically encouraged and placed in settings conducive to new, shared perspectives. It is important to keep in mind, however, that the frontiers of health care and education do not extend to the recesses of traditional practice. As we move beyond demonstration projects and voluntary collaborations to institutionalized reform and demands for change, the entire nature of the process is likely to shift. With it, predictions of rapid change are likely to be seen as premature and naïve. In addition, it is important to keep in mind that by no means do all the ferment and paradigm shifts within medicine and education lead either logically or pragmatically toward integration.

Although proceeding with integration of the medical and educational frameworks seems, on the surface, to be rather obvious and a simple thing to do, we do not believe that it is. Two programs have been initiated in the last eight to ten years, however, which reflect reasonably successful efforts by both health care and educational personnel to overcome the traditional barriers encountered: resistance to change, conservatism, inertia, and distrust of institutions and professionals.

The first to be described (Cambridge) develops a comprehensive health system for a target group of children under the auspices of the health institutions and locates it physically in the school building. The second to be described (Galveston), although in existence a slightly shorter period of time, was initiated from within an educational system with a tradition of school health dating back at least 50 years.

A MODEL: SCHOOL-BASED PRIMARY
HEALTH CARE IN CAMBRIDGE, MASSACHUSETTS

The Cambridge school-based primary care program for children operates under the auspices of the city's Department of Health and Hospital and is the immediate responsibility of the director of the Department of Pediatrics at the Cambridge Hospital, a city hospital. This structure places all municipal child health services under one administrative authority and brings coordination to previously fragmented programs.

Cambridge is a city independent of Boston with a population of 102,096 of whom 19,700 are children under 18 years of age. It has a heterogeneous population with respect to ethnic origin, race, educational levels, and socioeconomic status. Approximately 40 percent of its children seek private medical care. The remaining 60 percent reside primarily in the eastern and northern sections of the city. This population includes the majority of low income families who are increasingly dependent on municipal services for medical care as the number of family physicians steadily decreases. In 1975 approximately 13,800 children under 18 were living in the eastern and northern sections of the city— an area without the services of a practicing pediatrician.

The first primary care center for children opened in 1968, and four others have been established since that time. Four centers are located in elementary school health suites, and one is located in a building adjacent to the neighborhood school. The centers are open from 8:30 A.M. to 5:00 P.M., five days a week throughout the year, with weekend and night coverage provided by the pediatric staff of the Cambridge Hospital. Enrollment is open to any Cambridge child, and health center assignments are made on the basis of geographic convenience. One center remains open one evening a week to facilitate access for working mothers. Routine examinations are by appointment, although each health center accepts drop-in visits and also handles telephone consultations.

The program is designed so a child can be followed by a single integrated health service from birth through adolescence. The primary caretaker is the pediatric nurse practitioner who functions as case-finder, counselor, clinician, and patient advocate. Each center is staffed by two or three pediatric nurse practitioners and a health aide/translator. A senior pediatrician from the Department of Pediatrics at the Cambridge Hospital spends one-half day a week at each center. During this visit, the pediatrician sees children referred by the nurse practitioner for chronic problems not requiring acute hospital care and routinely examines all children at times specified by age.

The nurse practitioners are an integral part of the Department of Pediatrics. They participate regularly in all department rounds and conferences, consult with staff, visit admitted patients, and meet new mothers on the maternity floor. The hospital's pediatric ambulatory, inpatient, psychiatric, and social services are all closely coordinated with the health center system, providing a full range of services to children and families. The competence of the pediatric nurse practitioner has permitted a steady expansion of the program's scope to the point where a multiplicity of services are available. These services are designed to ensure that children receive medical care appropriate to their age and that parents receive appropriate education and support. The nurse practitioner has specific responsibilities in the areas of health maintenance, sick child care, school health, community outreach, and follow-up.

All Cambridge women who are delivered at the Cambridge Hospital are visited on the maternity floor by a nurse practitioner, and all Cambridge women who are delivered in other hospitals receive a home visit from a nurse practitioner soon after the birth certificate is registered in Cambridge. The purpose of these visits is to discuss infant care with the mother and to inform her of the services available in the program if she is without pediatric care. If the mother desires, an appointment is made at the nearest health center. The frequency of appointments is that recommended by the American Academy of Pediatrics, and each visit includes a physical examination by the nurse practitioner, age-appropriate immunizations, tuberculosis skin testing, hematocrits, blood lead determinations, hearing and vision screening, and developmental assessments.

In addition to her health maintenance responsibilities, the nurse practitioner also manages the minor illnesses and injuries of childhood under the supervision of a pediatrician. A senior staff pediatrician is available at all times for telephone consultation, and any child in need of immediate care is sent to the emergency ward at the Cambridge Hospital. For chronic conditions, the nurse practitioner can choose to have the child examined by the staff pediatrician at his weekly visit to the center.

The main thrust of the program for the school-age child is to identify as early as possible any child who is having difficulty adjusting to the classroom. Nurse practitioner/teacher conferences are held three times a year and serve as the means of identifying children with a learning disability or emotional difficulty. Upon identification of such a child, referrals are made to the Children's Developmental Clinic, which is part of the Department of Pediatrics. As remedial programs are developed, the nurse practitioner functions as the coordinator between school consultant, family, and child.

All enrolled children are given a thorough preschool evaluation by the nurse practitioner. Children in schools without a health center are examined by a school physician in the traditional manner or by their private pediatrician, and the examination is recorded on the school health record. Each public and parochial school in Cambridge receives school health services. Schools associated with the primary care program are covered by the center's nurse practitioners. The other schools are served by traditional school nurses who refer children, when appropriate, to the nearest health center or to their private physician.

In addition to newborn home visits, the nurse practitioners visit multiproblem families, families whose children have been seen in the emergency ward, and families who have repeatedly missed appointments. The nurse practitioners give consultation to the staffs of day care centers and nursery schools regarding communicable diseases, first aid, and nutrition. They also meet with parent groups regarding child rearing concerns and coordinate efforts with social welfare agencies concerning the management of multiproblem children and families.

During the eight years the school-based primary care program has been in operation, it has had a number of effects on child health services.

Results of the School-Based Primary Care Program

Comprehensive medical services have been made available to the community. Before establishment of the program, services to sick children were separate from well child care. The traditional Well Child Conferences were primarily immunization clinics; few children attended after two years of age. The school health program consisted of routine physical examinations by the school physicians at grades one, five, and nine. These examinations were cursory, and provisions for treatment and follow-up were lacking. Children now have the opportunity to receive all levels of care through a coordinated referral system.

A high level of penetration has been achieved in the eligible community—in 1975 the program reached 2,472 preschool children (77 percent of those eligible) and 3,500 school-age children (54 percent of the total elementary population of the city). There were 29,000 visits to the centers in 1975—20,000 visits by school children and 9,000 by preschoolers. For some areas, more than 90 percent of all geographically eligible children are enrolled at the appropriate center. The majority of nonenrolled children are seen by private pediatricians or in the health services of Harvard University or Massachusetts Institute of Technology. Presently, there is no significant group of Cambridge children without pediatric care.

The number of children entering school who are immunized for measles rose from 55 percent in 1965 to 99 percent in 1975. Ninety-eight percent of children entering school in the fall of 1975 had completed their DPT and polio series. This figure represents all Cambridge children.

Elevated blood levels of lead were found in seven percent of the centers' preschool population in 1973. A lead detection program was introduced, and in 1975, the incidence of elevated blood levels of lead was less than 0.5 percent.

A nutritional evaluation of the centers' populations revealed inadequate nutrition in a significant number of enrollees. WIC Supplemental Food Program funds (a federal program) were sought and obtained. Within one year, this program has been associated with a reduction in the rate of iron deficiency anemia in one- to two-year-olds from 16 percent to 4 percent and two- to three-year-olds from 22 percent to 7 percent.

Referral data from one center over a one-year period indicate that 78 percent of referrals made were completed. The majority of referrals were to the Department of Pediatrics at the Cambridge Hospital, 30 percent for recurrent ear disease, 12 percent for dermatologic conditions, 9 percent for surgical problems, and 41 percent for other medical reasons. The total number of referrals from all centers has remained fairly constant at four percent of patient visits.

Changes in utilization of existing medical facilities has occurred as a result of the program. One of the most striking changes was a change in the usage of the Cambridge Hospital Emergency Ward. Excessive use of the emergency room (ER) for routine pediatric care was documented in 1965. Pediatric emergency room utilization was restudied in 1973, after the primary care system had been established; and it was found that the number of appropriate ER visits increased significantly in the areas where health centers were present. There was no significant change in utilization for children from other areas of Cambridge, nor in a comparison group from an adjoining city without comprehensive child health services. Because the health centers meet the primary care needs of a large proportion of Cambridge children, the Pediatric Outpatient Department of the Cambridge Hospital has been able to shift its emphasis from health maintenance services to the provision of consultative care. The effective referral system from health center to hospital and hospital to health center has made it possible to provide services at an appropriate level.

The program has provided a realistic and challenging educational experience for house officers and students. In the course of a year, 21 first-year house officers, ten second-year, and six third-year officers rotate through the Department of Pediatrics from the Children's Service at the Massachusetts General Hospital. In addition, 48 medical students spend one month in the Department of Pediatrics, and for some it is their only exposure to pediatrics. Although the major assignment of the house officers and medical students is covering hospital functions, all spend time in the neighborhood health centers seeing patients with the nurse practitioners. The senior resident devotes 50 percent of his time to serving as a consultant to the nurse practitioners. Increasingly, this program is seen by students and house officers as a most valuable opportunity to become involved in primary care pediatrics in an academic setting.

Concurrent with the reorganization of child health services, a unique data collection system has been established to record changes in patient utilization and in medical services rendered in the health centers. The system uses prescored punch cards for information input and a set of computer programs for editing and recording data. Each nurse practitioner and health aide has a small card holder with a clear plastic template (IBM Port-A-Punch) in which the card is punched. All reportable information is punched daily by whoever provides the service. Cards are collected at a central location and sent monthly to a computer center for editing and generation of activity reports. The system is mechanically simple, easy to use, portable, and inexpensive, with no need for keypunchers or intermediate data handlers.

The program is cost-effective, as Table 3-1 indicates. The cost of the present clinical program represents no new monies expended by the city, state, or federal government. Reallocation of existing resources from the School Health Program and Well Child Conferences and the replacement of retiring school nurses and school physicians by pediatric nurse practitioners have resulted in the present comprehensive program, which actually costs less than the previously disjointed effort.

Table 3-1 Cost of Primary Care Program (1974)

Total number of Cambridge children	18,000
Number enrolled in primary care program	6,000
Number of primary care visits	28,228
Total cost of primary care (5 centers)	$210,900.00
Per capita cost per year	35.15
Cost per visit	7.47

This comprehensive program did not spring into being overnight but was developed gradually from existing municipal health programs. Before 1967 city health and hospital services were administered by separate departments. Inpatient, outpatient, and emergency services were located at the Cambridge Hospital, and the Health Department provided traditional well child and school health services, which were not closely coordinated to each other or to the pediatric services at the hospital. Each had separate records and different physicians and, therefore, tended to duplicate and fragment health care. Most of the children served by the Health Department's Well Child Conferences were under two years of age and were seen for immunizations, since there was no provision for care of the sick child. The School Health Program offered physical examinations by the school physician for children in the first, fifth, and ninth grades, but due to the periodic nature of the contact, these examinations did not provide an opportunity for the physician to become aware of the child's academic performance or emotional adjustment or to follow-up on any medical condition that was discovered. School nursing time was devoted primarily to first aid and record keeping, with limited amounts of time available for home visiting or follow-up of referrals.

In 1967 the Cambridge City Council passed an ordinance which established a combined Department of Health and Hospital to be administered by a commissioner. The commissioner assigned responsibility for all child health services of the health department to the director of pediatrics at the Cambridge Hospital. The director began at that time to develop the integrated municipal child health program that is described above. In addition to the municipal services, two other public child health programs under separate administrations were added to the system. They were the health services of the city's Head Start Program and of a remedial education program under the Office of Education called Follow Through.

Before the first health center was established surveys of existing health resources and of patterns of utilization were done. Both of these studies indicated that specific geographic areas in the eastern and northern sections of Cambridge were most in need of child health services. In 1965 there were 14 practicing physicians serving this population, and only one was a pediatrician, who has since retired. Their mean age was 57 years. No new physicians had entered practice in the previous decade, and it seemed unlikely that any would in the near future. A majority of Cambridge physicians who were interviewed during these early planning stages indicated that they were not serving this pediatric population and voiced support for a future program that would insure the availability of high quality, cost-effective pediatric care to all Cambridge families.

At the same time, an analysis of the pediatric population using the Cambridge Hospital Emergency Ward revealed that this facility was serving as family physician for a large number of patients residing in the densely populated areas in the eastern and northern sections of the city. Seventy percent of the emergency ward diagnoses were for upper respiratory infections and minor injuries. One community in the eastern section of the city was selected as being in particular need. This area contained the city's largest public housing project, the highest prematurity rate, and the greatest density of children. Within this community lived 2,100 children under the age of 18 years; 550 were preschoolers. In addition, community leadership was strong and interest in providing new services was high. A task force of community leaders was established to assist in the planning; and, after two years of meetings, support had been developed for the concept of delivery of primary care by a group of pediatric nurse practitioners who were school-based.

The task force was initiated because of the mutual concern of the director of pediatrics and community leaders regarding the quality of available child health services. The meetings were scheduled by parents and held in multiple sites throughout the city (churches, community centers, and homes). The agenda remained constant and consisted of the community's critique of the existing system and their expression of the ideal program. There were difficult local issues; that is, each neighborhood felt that its need was paramount and that if a new service were to be instituted, it should be instituted there first. An ever-increasing number of parents became involved during the two years, which gave the meetings an unstructured format. Realistic alternatives, however, evolved from the discussions.

The public health nurses employed by the city, whose primary responsibility was to function in the Well Child and School Health Program, were offered an opportunity to enroll in a Pediatric Nurse Practitioner training program. A few were interested at the outset, and three attended the course. Only one functioned in the practitioner role and subsequently decided to revert to the traditional school nurse role. As school nurses retired, nurse practitioners were hired to staff the evolving system of health centers.

In July 1968 the first center opened. Clinical efforts were focused on providing physical examinations and routine services to preschool children. Outreach efforts were directed toward mothers of young children, informing them of the availability of primary care at the center.

A firm relationship with the community had been established, and the service quickly evolved toward the model described above.

Subsequent to the opening of the initial center, two new elementary schools were constructed in the eastern section of the city. The director of pediatrics worked with the school architect and the superintendent of schools in developing ample space for health services in these new buildings. In two other elementary schools, existing school health suites were already suitable to house the expanding services. The superintendent of schools and the director of pediatrics developed a working relationship following a series of discussions regarding the total needs of Cambridge children. The superintendent was supportive of the concept of broadening the school health program to one that included primary care services and was enthusiastic that this effort be school-based. Subsequent superintendents have all had a commitment to an expanded school health program. The relationship between the pediatric nurse practitioners and the school department has become a closer one over the years, largely because school personnel have come to understand the advantages of having an expanded clinical service available to students.

By 1972 five centers were created, and by 1976 the five school-based health centers were well established and providing primary pediatric care as well as accessibility to a comprehensive health care system. Attention is now being given to the development of an adolescent program based in the high school and coordinating this program with the existing effort.

PUBLIC SCHOOL HEALTH SERVICES IN GALVESTON, TEXAS: A MODEL FOR CHANGE

The community of Galveston has long recognized the importance of providing for the health care of school children, both within the school setting and through the facilities of primary care providers. The community has benefited by the presence of a large medical school, the University of Texas Medical Branch. School board-appointed school nurses, with medical and dental consultation available, have been in the public schools for more than 50 years. Today, Galveston's school health program includes many new and innovative ideas that have led to new approaches to health services and education. How was change brought about? What process took place?

The Health Services Department of the Galveston Independent School District operates under the auspices of the Board of Trustees. The board has adopted certain statements that reflect its goals, and these statements form the basis of the philosophy of the health program. The goals are to promote the overall well-being and optimal future functioning in society of every Galveston child.

Administratively, a pediatric medical director and a nursing coordinator of school health services report directly to an assistant superintendent. The medical director may consult, however, with anyone in the school district. All nurses are employed by the Board of Trustees.

Community

Galveston is an island city located off the Texas coast in the Gulf of Mexico. The population is approximately 64,000, of whom 20,000 are children under 18 years of age (1970 federal census). The Galveston Independent School District (GISD) has a membership of approximately 10,000 students attending one large high school, four middle schools, nine elementary schools, a secondary guidance center, an early childhood learning center, and a sheltered workshop for the mentally retarded. About 2,000 children are enrolled in private or parochial schools on the island. In the public elementary schools in Galveston, the ethnic distribution is 42 percent Negro-American, 35 percent Anglo-American, and 23 percent Mexican-American. The family distribution by Hollinghead's index of socioeconomic level is 3 percent upper, 2 percent upper middle, 13 percent middle, 36 percent lower middle, and 46 percent lower. Ten school nurses are employed (approximately one per 1,000 students), eight of whom are pediatric nurse practitioners. Many resources are avaialble for health care on the island, including general and specialist private practitioners, the University of Texas Medical Branch (UTMB) facilities, the University of Texas School of Nursing, the Health Department, and many social and welfare agencies.

Background

Prior to 1970, aside from a relatively good ratio of school nurses to students (about 1:1,000), the school health services were traditional. The major programs were first aid and vision and hearing screening. An unusual feature was the long-time existence of a dental clinic in one of the middle schools in a geographic area of high need. The Children and Youth Project assumed major financial responsibility for the staffing of this facility in 1967.

Development of the Program and Major Features

In 1970, on the retirement of the part-time school physician, a collaborative relationship between the medical school and the public school system was initiated. This occurred as a result of the superintendent's interest in a role for the schools that would extend some of their activities into health and social welfare spheres, thus enabling the schools to better meet the educational needs of an economically deprived population. The medical school pediatric department was also interested in developing community and school health programs to explore the boundary areas of child health care and advocacy. A pediatrician from the Department of Pediatrics was appointed medical director; and, at the same time, a coordinator of GISD Health Services was appointed who had broad experience in school and public health nursing.

Initial planning included an evaluation of existing programs and services and subsequent development of a three-year plan of improvement by using existing staff and resources. Staff nurses were asked to keep a record of their duties for a two-week period. After this time, they assigned these activities to one of two categories—those which, in their opinion, required professional training and those which, in their opinion, could be performed by less trained but supervised aides. The staff concluded that an expanded nurse's role would be desirable.

In 1970 and 1971 the availability of demonstration projects in school health (the Health and Nutrition Projects funded by the U.S. Office of Education) gave an opportunity to develop further a comprehensive school health plan and to extend the initial three-year plan to a five- and then seven-year projection. Since the projects were to focus on economically disadvantaged school children, five of the elementary school attendance zones were chosen as target schools. A profile of these schools revealed low immunization levels, poor nutritional status (as determined by a national survey), and lower academic achievement levels. The use of existing community health and social services was low, the completion of recommended referrals after school health assessments was low, and absenteeism rates were high.

A parental advisory committee, convened to assist in preparation of the grant application, confirmed the needs previously identified. They also suggested that an active outreach program be developed in the form of Home-School Agents who could establish a better relationship between the schools and the parents in the neighborhood. It was believed that much of the failure to utilize community services was due to a lack of knowledge and skill in getting access to the services and using them.

The project was then developed to address the above issues: a shared medical record and outreach workers to bridge the gap between the school, family, and community services; health aides to take over some of the clerical and first-aid duties of the nurse; nutritional education programs; and additional dental services through the university's Children and Youth Project (C&Y). Each child enrolled in the project had, through the C&Y Project, complete screening history, physical and laboratory examinations including tuberculin skin test, immunization check, complete blood count, urinalysis, urine culture, height and weight. Problem areas identified were worked on by the team—health aide, nurse, and home-school agent. Parent groups were organized and community education undertaken with the valuable assistance of the home-school agents.

Developing the Expanded Nurse Role

Between 1971 and 1973 the project, funded for these service functions, continued with good local support and additional principals requesting the program's services in their schools. While the need for an expanded nursing role continued to be apparent, no local resources existed for pediatric nurse practitioner (PNP) training. The medical director then took a brief sabbatical experience with Henry Silver in Denver, Colorado. Upon his return, the nursing school was successful in initiating this resource for PNP training in Galveston in 1973. This resource, plus support from the Texas Regional Medical Program and the commitment of the Board of Education, allowed for the beginning of the transition of the school nursing staff to become pediatric nurse practitioners and apply these skills to their school nursing activities.

Implementation of the role of the pediatric nurse practitioner as a school nurse required several facilitating activities. One was the identification of physician preceptors and back-ups who could be in the school initially on a one-half day per week basis when the school PNP was returning to develop the new role. Over the years, this interdependent role was developed between nurses and university pediatric fellows, residents, faculty members, and private practitioners in the community. A workshop, meeting twice monthly during the school year, discussed topics and approaches to case management.

Another important initiating factor in an expanded role was a series of rap sessions between the nurses and the principals led by an anthropologist from the university. During these sessions nurses' duties and principals' expectations were openly and frankly discussed with better appreciation of the needs and pressures on both groups.

The third important initiating factor was the administrative support and direction-setting toward this expanded nurse role. Both nursing and medical leaders were careful to involve and solicit the support of key school administrators and school board members. An important commitment to the expanded nurse role was achieved when the school board voted to guarantee the positions of those who took the additional training by assuring that they would be placed on local funds if grant monies were no longer available to pay them. They also agreed to a small financial incentive to be paid to nurses who returned from successfully completing PNP training.

Further Collaborative Efforts

In 1973, as a result of the successful interaction between GISD and UTMB, a School Health Programs Advisory Committee was established. This committee was set up because the university was interested in coordinating and further developing community school health programs. Participating in this effort were representatives from pediatrics, psychiatry, nursing, preventive medicine, ob-gyn, and the local school systems. A new medical director was recruited for the faculty, one who had special interests and training in school health.

An area of need identified at this time was support for continuation of the development of a comprehensive school health program and support for an evaluation of the impact of the attempt to link school and primary health care services. This need was met in 1974 when a five-year project grant was approved by The Robert Wood Johnson Foundation.

The purpose of that project was to build on the existing program in the following manner: to continue and to evaluate the demonstration of this new model of school health services; to develop further the application of a computer-operated health information system; to train physicians, nurses, allied professionals, and educators in the principles and practice of child and school health; and to develop some new approaches to health education. The Health Information System has grown from its initial goal of facilitating feedback and communication between the school and UTMB to a management system for health information for all children seen at the UTMB Department of Pediatrics. Currently, automatic processing results in periodic reports to school nurses on children whose parents have granted permission for sharing of information to both institutions.

Physician activities in school health have included medical consultation on school health policies, practices, and reassessment of screening procedures (dropping urine cultures and nonproductive lab screening), and adding scoliosis screening and physical therapy consultation. Back-up for PNPs includes supervising required physical examination forms for special education students and establishing standing orders for the treatment of pediculosis (head lice). Physicians have also provided in-service education for teachers and other school staff, served on pupil assessment teams for children with learning or behavioral problems, served as resources for target health education programs (obesity, asthma, sex education), and acted as a liaison to sources of primary and secondary health care services in Galveston.

Health Education Demonstration Activities

The Galveston Independent School District and the School Health Programs of the University of Texas Medical Branch have been working together to demonstrate new approaches to health education in the schools. The major purposes for the activities were to reach a large number of school personnel to increase interest in developing health education programs, to develop a structured and carefully evaluated health education program that can demonstrate impact on children's health, and to involve education and health professionals in working together to plan and carry out health education programs.

Health Skills for Kindergarten Children

The skills approach to health education was used as the conceptual framework for developing the program. The learning activities were structured around skills the children could develop for health-related behavior. The three skills identified for the program were that children would be able to identify and express to adults feelings of illness and wellness, to identify appropriate sources of assistance for health problems, and to initiate by themselves the use of sources for assistance for health-related problems. These skills were judged to be appropriate for the developmental level of kindergarten children and to initiate the reinforcement of an internal locus of control regarding health behavior.

The program consisted of four sequential lessons plus suggested learning activities to provide additional opportunities for children to practice skills. The first lesson involved medical students visiting the classrooms and talking with the children about what it means to be healthy or sick, what they can do when they feel sick, and how the doctor, nurse, or other adults can help children when they are sick. The remaining lessons included a clarification of feelings and how feelings can be expressed, ways in which illness influences one's actions and feelings, and what children can do and who can help when they feel sick.

Some of the lessons utilize materials and activities from the published affective education program titled Development of Understanding of Self and Others (DUSO).[14] The reason for using the DUSO material was to familiarize teachers with the program with the hope that more teachers would incorporate DUSO activities into their teaching.

Health Education Program for Children with Asthma

The program for asthmatic children was developed to demonstrate a model for health education that focuses on a target population with identified health needs. Children with asthma were selected as a target group to evaluate a school-based health education program jointly planned and conducted by health and educational personnel. Asthmatic children were selected because they constitute the largest group of school-age children with a single chronic condition, and there is some limited evidence that special educational programs for asthmatics have contributed to an improvement in their health status.

The overall educational goals of the program are to assist children in understanding their asthmatic condition and to help them assume greater responsibility and involvement in the management of their asthma. Specific objectives for the children participating in the program are a reduction in the number of asthma attacks requiring emergency medical treatment, a decrease in the number of school days missed, a reduction in the level of anxiety associated with illness, an improvement in attitudes toward self, an improvement in perception of self-control for health behavior, and an increase in children's and parents' knowledge of asthma and management procedures.

The pilot phase of the project involved one elementary school (grades kindergarten to five). A health educator from the Department of Pediatrics and the school pediatric nurse practitioner conducted weekly 40-minute sessions for seven months of the school year. Thirteen children participated in the program in two different age groups (grades K-2 and 3-5). Structured lessons were developed and piloted to assist the children in understanding concepts related to the nature of asthma, the causes of attacks, and prevention and treatment measures. Lessons also dealt with decision making and feelings about asthma. In addition, a published, structured program in affective education (*Dimensions of Personality*) was used to assist children in learning about themselves and for reinforcing positive attitudes toward self.

A pediatric allergist and a school social worker offered parents an opportunity to meet to learn about asthma and discuss some of their concerns about having an asthmatic child. Parent meetings were poorly attended and eventually were dropped from the program. One exception to the poor attendance was a family evening when the children showed their parents a television tape of their classes and examples of their learning activities. Almost all the mothers and one father attended this meeting and participated in teaching the children breathing exercises.

Following the pilot, the program was revised and plans made to phase the program into all elementary schools over a two-year period. This allowed time for training of personnel and a means of establishing an evaluation design that provided a treatment and a comparison group of asthmatic children. To give the program a broader base of support in the school and to tap the skills of other professionals, the approach to staffing the program was changed to a "program team." The first year the team consisted of the school nurse, the school physician or a community physician consultant, school psychologist, resource teacher or classroom teacher, and the physical education teacher. In the second year of the project, special education personnel (school psychologist and resource teachers) were not involved in those schools providing the health education program.

An outcome of the project was the development of a patient education book for children with asthma. It is titled *Teaching My Parents About Asthma* and is designed to develop five skill areas that are applied to self-care for asthma.[15] These include being able to observe situations that might lead to an asthma attack (observation skills); being able to notice changes that would indicate a pending or actual asthma attack (discrimination skills); being able to make decisions to take action themselves or to get help to prevent or stop an asthma attack (decision-making skills); being able to tell parents, doctors, or others what is happening to them just before and during an asthma attack (communication skills); and maintaining a strong positive attitude about being able to do things to help themselves with asthma (self-reliance). The book includes information and learning experiences for the children on the right side of the page and, on the left side, more detailed information for parents, as well as suggested activities for helping the child learn and develop skills. The book provides an alternative means of encouraging parental involvement and reinforcement for the children. For the children in grades three, four, and five, the book provides the structure for the group teaching. In the lower grades, stories based on the concepts in the book are used to provide the structure. The learning activities are designed to demonstrate a model for applying the skills approach to health education for target groups of children with common health needs.

Adolescent Health Survey

To facilitate the planning of health programs for adolescents in Galveston, a survey was conducted to determine perceived health needs. A self-administered anonymous questionnaire was completed by 3,255 of 3,874 Galveston high school students. The results of the survey indicated that all aspects of health (concerns, perceived adequacy of knowledge, problems, sources of care, and utilization of health care resources) were significantly influenced by the ethnic background, grade level, or sex of the surveyed high school students.

The most striking differences were found in the use of different health care resources. Regardless of socioeconomic status, black students relied more on public health facilities than whites, who tended to go to private doctors. Although Mexican-American students had the highest proportion in the lowest socioeconomic levels, they were less likely to use public health facilities. Mexican-American students gave less consideration to health matters than did the other two ethnic groups, and lower proportions reported a need for information, identified problems requiring help, or reported thinking often about their health. As a group, however, they had the lowest proportion rating their health as very good and the highest reporting that they did not get answers to questions about health because no one was available to ask.

Girls were more likely than boys to identify problems requiring assistance. Information or assistance with sexually related problems was expressed as more of a need by girls than by boys. As students became older, they were more likely to identify the need for assistance with health problems. The younger students either had fewer problems or were less likely to be aware of their needs with regard to some problem areas. There is an exception to this age trend with drinking and drug use. The youngest students were more likely to express the need for assistance with drinking and drug use; that need appears to decrease with age.

Students appear to be able to select appropriate community sources for dealing with specific problems. Resources available in the school, however, were infrequently selected as a source for dealing with specific problems. The highest ranked concerns and problems were school, drugs, sex, getting along with parents and adults, acne, depression, and overweight. Ninety-one percent reported they often or sometimes worry about their health. Sources of medical care were family doctor (56.8 percent) and hospital emergency room (15.9 percent). Reported visits to a doctor in the past year: none (27.5 percent); one (24.1 percent); two to three (32.2 percent; and four or more (14.7 percent).

In analyzing responses according to sex, grade, and ethnic background, several implications are apparent: many of the concerns and problems identified require educational as well as health care services; the diverse perceived health needs of an entire high school population indicate that the traditional one-semester general health course for all is grossly inadequate; and students' concerns and problems are not limited to the areas of drugs, venereal disease, and birth control.

One of the outcomes of the adolescent health survey was the formation of a planning group at the high school. Members of the group have agreed to work collectively toward developing activities or programs that would address some of the needs identified through the survey. Thus far the group includes students, teachers, counselors, a school social worker, a school nurse, a school physician, and a health educator. The next step also is to form a community group of individuals interested in adolescent health needs. This group would function to develop programs and activities outside the school and would also work with the school group to coordinate activities and provide resources for school programs.

The primary goal of both groups is to provide health education and services that are based on identified student needs and are individualized to the point of meeting the great diversity of health-related concerns or problems. The experience gained through this demonstration project emphasizes the need for cooperative planning between school and community personnel as well as the need for joint programs involving health services and educational professionals working together.

Sex Education for Adolescents

The adolescent health survey confirmed the subjective impression of educational and health personnel that there is a need for educational programs to help adolescents understand and deal with their sexuality. Prior to program development in sex education, the UTMB School Health Programs organized an interdisciplinary planning committee at the university. The committee developed and conducted a pilot sex education course for adolescents ages 11 to 14 years. The course consisted of eight 90-minute sessions that included the presentation of information as well as small group discussions. The first pilot course was conducted in the evening on the university campus.

As a result of the pilot course, the Parent-Teacher's Association (PTA) at one of the middle schools in Galveston became interested in providing a similar program for eighth grade students. Two planning committees were established, one at the school and one at UTMB. The school committee accomplished the planning for scheduling, gaining school personnel support, informing parents and students about the program, and involving some teachers as group leaders in teaching the course. The university committee planned the course curriculum, evaluation procedures, and in-service training for course group leaders.

The course was conducted as an after-school program held once a week for eight weeks. Approximately 50 students participated. As a result of the first year's experience, interest, and support have been generated to continue the development of sex education programs that would involve cooperative efforts of community, school, and medical center personnel.

Impact of the Project

Before the initiation of the efforts described above, the only data available on the outcome of referrals for identified problems indicate that about 41 percent of such referrals reached care. For the 1976—77 school year, 82 percent of all referrals received care: 89 percent for physical examinations, 100 percent for immunizations, 90 percent for trauma, 68 percent for dental,* 61 percent for visual acuity, 75 percent for hearing acuity, and 89 percent for other medical referrals.

During the Health and Nutrition Project, a ten percent subsample of children was repeatedly examined each year for the three project years. Analysis of the problems found indicated that each year the number of children with uncorrected health problems and multiple health problems decreased.

In one of the high school clinics, a nurse compared her experience before and after she received the PNP training. During comparable time periods roughly the same number of school clinic visits (3,450) were made by students. The number of problems identified as requiring outside referral, however, increased from 60 in the year before PNP training (1973–74) to 132 in the following year. Also, the percentage who reached a source of care increased from 50 percent to 86 percent. Nurse contact with other health care providers also increased from five contacts to 22 contacts.

About 45 percent of school children had been immunized in 1971 when a statewide compulsory immunization law was introduced. This had increased to 99 percent by June 1976.

A current evaluation protocol was initiated in 1977 as a joint effort of the university and the school system. It will document episodes of health care for a random sample of elementary school children. The role of the school will be documented in initiating access to the health care system and in noting in what way the school facilitates the ongoing care for acute and chronic illnesses and health maintenance activities. Which children in the community benefit most from the expanded school services will be noted, and indices of the overall functioning of the school health program will be derived. In addition, repeated task analyses of school nurse activities will document any changes which take place.

---

*Dental—68% referral completion for the 1975—76 school year.

The efforts spent in developing and implementing the described school health program have resulted in several papers and descriptions of project activities.[16-23] Staff members have been an integral part of the process that led to the program in effect today. Participants are aware that change is constant and that tomorrow better ideas will replace those accepted as good today.

CONCLUSION

The reader might question the present level of success in the two models cited in truly integrating the educational and health institutions to meet specific health or educational needs of children, but only time and further study will determine whether the program made a difference in the health and functioning of children. At the heart of the problem of integrating schools and health care is the existence of deeply held but usually unacknowledged models of work and values that are partially in fundamental conflict (see Table 3-2).

An exploration of the medical and the educational frameworks suggests that their divergence, partial overlap, and mutual deficiencies are substantial factors in establishing innovative school health programs. For example, nurses with expanded skills are often seen as the central figure in models for change. Our analysis would suggest, however, that their effectiveness could continue to be undercut if the larger medical care system does not accept a redefinition of professional roles and if

Table 3-2 Potential Conflicts in Approach Between School and Health Frameworks

Health Framework	School Framework
1. Child is of interest because he has a disease or problem that can be cured or ameliorated: therapy	1. Child is of interest because he has potential to learn or perform with peers: socialization
2. Goal is to identify pathology and rehabilitate, ameliorate, or cure	2. Goal is to elicit and demonstrate "normality" or excellence
3. Encounters are episodic and individual, out of natural context	3. Encounters are in groups, sustained and routinized
4. Approach is relatively impersonal, scientific or "case management" oriented	4. Approach is highly interpersonal, contextualized, and relatively intuitive
5. Expectation is of professional control of conditions of work	5. Expectation is of (if not pleasure at) public, bureaucratic control of conditions of work
6. Power is self-assured, as profession	6. Power is defensive, as partial profession

school personnel do not learn how to work with the PNP in new ways. True integration and expansion of the models will be difficult and time-consuming; it will mean that everyone involved will have to give up some traditional ways of viewing the child, their own work, and the work of others. We have raised more questions than have been answered. The answers must come from us all.

REFERENCES

1. P. W. Jackson, *Life in Classrooms* (New York: Holt, Rinehart and Winston, 1968), p. 149.

2. D. C. Lortie, *Schoolteacher: A Sociological Study* (Chicago: University of Chicago Press, 1975).

3. Children's Defense Fund of the Washington Research Project, *Children Out of School In America* (October 1974). Publisher: Children's Defense Fund, Washington, D.C.

4. Lortie, *op. cit.*, p. 114.

5. A. B. Ford, R. E. Liske, R. S. Ort, and J. C. Denton, *The Doctor's Perspective: Physicians View Their Patients and Practice* (Cleveland: The Press of Case Western Reserve University, 1967), p. 144.

6. Jackson, *op. cit.*, p. 171.

7. E. Freidson, *Profession of Medicine: A Study of the Sociology of Applied Knowledge* (New York: Dodd, Mead and Company, 1972).

8. Lortie, *op. cit.*

9. *Ibid.*, pp. 22-23.

10. Jackson, *op. cit.*

11. M. Meyer, "Teacher Training," in Bernard Johnston, Ed., *Issues in Education: An Anthology of Controversy* (Boston: Houghton-Mifflin, 1964).

12. Lortie, *op. cit.*; H. S. Becker, B. Geer, B. C. Hughes, and A. L. Strauss, *Boys in White: Student Culture in Medical School* (Chicago: University of Chicago Press, 1961); R. K. Merton, G. G. Reeder, and P. L. Kendall, Eds., *The Student-Physician* (Cambridge, Mass: Harvard University Press, 1957).

13. Lortie, *op. cit.*, p. 186.

14. D. Dinkmeyer, *Developing Understanding of Self and Others* (Circle Pines, Minn.: American Guidance Service, 1970).

15. G. S. Parcel, K. Tiernan, P. R. Nader, and L. Weiner, *Teaching My Parents About Asthma* (Galveston, Texas: Department of Pediatrics, University of Texas Medical Branch, 1976).

16. J. Conrad, "The High School Nurse as a Pediatric Nurse Practitioner," *Pediatric Nursing* no. 6 (Nov. 1975): 15-17.

17. R. McKevitt, P. R. Nader, M. Williamson, and R. Berrey, "Reasons for Health Office Visits in an Urban School District," *Journal of School Health* 47, no. 5 (1977): 275.

18. "The Whole Child. Based on Interviews with P. R. Nader and J. Conrad," in *Casebook of Physician-Nurse Joint Practices in Primary Care* (Chicago: Educational Publications and Innovative Communications, 1976).

19. School Health Programs and Galveston Independent School District: *School Health: A Model for Change* (Galveston, Texas: University of Texas Medical Branch, 1974) (videotape, color, 31 min.).

20. *School Health Programs Newsletter*. A monthly publication from the School Health Programs, University of Texas Medical Branch, distributed nationally. Available from School Health Programs, 1202 Market Street, Galveston, Texas 77550.

21. G. Parcel, P.R. Nader, and M. Meyer, "Assessing Adolescent Health Concerns, Problems and Patterns of Utilization in a Triethnic Urban Population," *Pediatrics* 60, No. 2 (Aug. 1977): 157.

22. P. R. Nader, "The University Medical Center and School Health," presented at American Public Health Association, New Orleans, Louisiana, October 1974.

23. G. S. Parcel, "The University Medical Center and School Health: Implications for School Health Education," presented at American Public Health Association, New Orleans, Louisiana, October 1974.

Chapter 4

From Plan to Practice: The Process of Achieving a Successful School Health Program

Elizabeth Bryan, M.D., and
John G. Bruhn, Ph.D.

Although the health and education of students are of concern in every community, the priority of the concern and the degree of compromise in differing viewpoints will determine whether there is a school health program, and, if one exists, its quality and effectiveness. Whatever the goals, school health requires teamwork from plan to practice. In this chapter, we will identify the steps, strategies, and specific details in the process of "doing" school health that communities need to know as they plan their school health programs.

BACKGROUND

Forces Behind a Plan

School health is a community affair, so it involves the interplay among ideas, needs, and priorities of all the institutions, organizations, and members of a community. For a school health program to happen, a community must indicate some degree of support. Although the health and education of students are usually of great concern to persons in the community and often elicit strong reactions, school health will not always be ranked high in their actual priorities. Furthermore, school health can rise or fall in the priority rankings as the needs of communities change over time. It is important, therefore, to know one's own community to know its ideas about school health and its priority. Viewed this way, school health is an integral part of the total community system.

59

It is tempting to isolate the ideas and priorities of three components of a community system (that is, the school, health professionals, and parents) in deciding whether to plan a school health program. The school recognizes that how well students learn is related to how healthy they are; health professionals know that students are nowhere as healthy as they could be; and parents, although concerned about their children's health, find it almost impossible to participate in health decisions or to take initiatives regarding health that affect them and their children. Each of these components has a vested interest in the health and education of students and, thus, could be a strong advocate for a school health program. An effective and efficient school health program must also have the support of community agencies, health practitioners, clinics, and hospitals. It is necessary to consider the possibility of linking the various parts of the social system in the process by which school health can emerge as a priority in a community.

R. J. Haggerty has postulated four perceived options for school health:[1]

1. Medicine should not become involved in school health. Selection of this option would restrict physicians and health professionals to involvement with the health of students outside the school. Students would be brought to physicians to have problems treated, often after the episode has become more serious and complex. This option would downgrade prevention, would be expensive, would create a dependence on medicine, would create a danger of "overmedicalizing" the health problem, and would advocate the model of curative medicine.

2. School to deliver traditional health services. This option would use the school as the primary site for providing health services. Schools would have to increase the number of personnel and provide the necessary equipment and in-service education for teachers to handle a broad range of services. This would involve districtwide health services, which would exacerbate problems in communication, referral, and other areas. In addition, it would be difficult to involve parents in this approach, especially since they would be confused about when to use school-based versus nonschool-based health services.

3. School used as a site for health education. This option would encourage schools to include education about health in the total learning process. Education would include designs for healthful living. The Athenian school, a private, residential school in California, provides a model for discovery learning where students are ac-

quainted with real problems and issues as part of the learning about a particular subject. In this option, however, schools would have to revise curricula to include health and would have to employ health educators who could assume a major responsibility for teaching or could assemble teams appropriately trained to teach health.

4. Collaboration of teams to deal with learning and school problems. This option would utilize resources in the total community in such a manner that teams composed of representatives from disciplines would be assembled to deal with particular problems as they arise. Understanding and teamwork among the disciplines would be essential. The student and his problem would be the focus, rather than having the health services organized for the convenience of health professionals.

Obviously, each community has to weigh the efficacy and efficiency of these various options. Indeed, other options, as well as combinations of the above, are also possibilities. An option taken at one time may be substituted by another as circumstances and needs change. Perhaps the ideal option for school health is a plan or approach of "doing it together." The priority for school health should not be placed in an adversary or competitor position with priorities of other groups in the community. If school health programming is engaged in for purposes other than improving comprehensive health services for students, then school health programs become political tools, and funding and support for them become unpredictable. Too often, school health programs are planned segmentally with the aim of evolving a total plan as funds permit. A more effective approach is to design a total plan of phased implementation.

What School Health Can and Cannot Do

The goals and objectives of school health must be realistic. If parents expect the schools to assume health initiatives for them and their children, if educators feel that health professionals are telling them what to teach, and if health professionals feel that they are not asked to help plan or teach in health courses, students will become the pawns for rivalry and interprofessional jealousies. G. L. McAndrew has phrased the expectations regarding school health as follows:[2] if your approach is from the viewpoint of the learning of children, that is, their basic competency, you set the priorities for everybody; if you define what it is the children should learn, you define what the health people ought to be doing.

Perhaps the key point to be considered is that school health cannot do everything. If goals and objectives are too broad and idealistic, the schools, health professionals, and parents will be disappointed. The success or failure of a school health program is written, knowingly or unknowingly, as part of the plan.

The Change Agent

The generation of ideas, or the stimulation of people to think about needs and priorities, is usually precipitated by a change agent. This agent can be an individual or a group of varying size. The degree of success in mobilizing the community to a point of action depends on the strategy used. The several possible strategies include a community approach, self-help, problem-solving, demonstration, experimental, or power-conflict.[3] The approach to community organization that is used will depend on many factors, such as the size and nature of the community. With respect to formulating a plan for a school health program, the involvement of parents from the onset would enhance their later participation and support. No school health program can succeed without the broad support of parents. Support from selected parents, such as those who attend PTA meetings, can raise false hopes of broadening parental support once the program is initiated. Therefore, the initiators of change should not ignore the silent or nonparticipative segments of the community in the early stages of evolving a philosophy and plan for school health.

A Plan Needs Goals and Objectives

A school health program should have short, intermediate, and long-term goals. Later implementation and evaluation of program goals will be easier if goals are categorized in time increments. By employing an incremental approach, accomplishments can be easily and readily identified. This is of particular importance because the school, health professionals, and parents, as well as the rest of the community, will have periodic evidence of progress and will be more likely to give continued support to the program.

Other advantages to this method are that program activities and resources needed to accomplish these activities can be clearly identified, which will assist in the delineation of responsibilities, functions, and duties for personnel. In addition, it will be possible at any time to determine the progress being made in obtaining the planned program goals. Finally, program components can be easily identified and additions, modifications, or deletions can be made to suit changing conditions.

Goals determine objectives. Objectives are milestones along the way toward achieving goals—they are barometers to measure how well the goals are being met. In considering who should set goals and objectives for school health programs, it is important to sample the expectations regarding goals and objectives from as wide a range of the community as possible; but ultimately, goals and objectives must be limited to those that are realistically obtainable. This means that a small working group, composed of representatives from the school, the health professions, and the parents, must be involved in the final stages of evolving a school health plan.

Translating Objectives into Program

Objectives form the basis for designing programs. It is tempting to initiate programs first and then to seek objectives to justify the program. But programs that have no objectives usually have many difficulties. Personnel have neither common goals nor a clear idea of what they are working to accomplish, recipients do not have an understanding of what is expected of them, and funding problems usually develop, since guidelines for expending funds are not derived from specific goals and objectives.

Objectives can change for several reasons once a program is initiated. The program directors might find that the original objectives are too unrealistic, given the constraints discovered after the program was initiated. Thus, objectives may have to be scaled down in scope and in amount of time to accomplish them. Programs can also unintentionally stray from original objectives, as sometimes alternative objectives seem more interesting or appear more achievable once a program is started.

To alter programs for these reasons, however, reflects unfavorably on the planning process. It is advantageous to have explored as many of the obstacles to achievement of goals as possible before a program is initiated. Anticipation of problems with some thought to their possible solution will be helpful in seeking long-term support or funding.

Objectives should be practical and realistic. In the case of school health programs, objectives must have meaning to teachers, administrators, parents, and students. Objectives for school health programs must be geared to meeting the needs of students. Since the needs of students change, objectives should be realistic with respect to what can be achieved and how long it can be expected to take to achieve them. Parents will judge the importance or relevance of a program by whether it benefits their child at the time he or she is in school. Indeed, parents will often evaluate the importance of a program by whether their child is a participant in the program. Parents often object to letting their children participate in a program, such as a research project, where there is no direct or immediate benefit from participating.

Objectives should be clearly stated in terms understandable by all parties involved. Perhaps one of the most difficult tasks is to derive objectives for school health which have meaning across disciplines. It is difficult to elicit participation in a program if the objectives are not clear. School health is a multidisciplinary endeavor and objectives should have meaning to all personnel working in school health programs. If objectives are not free from jargon or are viewed as the objectives of only one discipline, territoriality and professional jealousies will be the downfall of the program. Thus, all parties who are to participate in a school health program should be involved in formulating objectives.

Objectives should be measurable. If they are not measurable through evaluation techniques, there is no way to determine the degree of success or failure of a program. Evaluation will be the key to deciding on the future scope and funding of a program. Programs often fail because they are guided by philosophic objectives that have no end point, or they can continue endlessly because no one has a clear idea of when the objective is accomplished. Such programs are often viewed as successes whether they fail or succeed, because there are no objective criteria to guide an evaluation of the effects of the program. The vested interests of program designers and benefits received by the recipients usually do not allow either to provide other than a glowing evaluation of the program.

Objectives should be incremental. It might take time to reach the final goal of a program; everyone needs a periodic assessment of how well he or she is doing. Program objectives need to be designed so progress can be assessed along the way. Thus, all parties will have periodic feedback on how far the program has moved and how far it has to go.

Objectives should have some degree of flexibility built into them so they can survive changes in policy and personnel. Sometimes program objectives are formulated around certain individuals who are known to be successful; and if those individuals should leave, objectives are viewed as not readily achievable. Programs are also begun under the sponsorship of one group of administrators who might change, and the new leadership might evaluate the program differently. This points up the need for a continual evaluation and feedback throughout a project so rational decisions can be made on available data.

Barriers in Planning Goals and Objectives

Effective advocacy for starting or changing a school health program involves being able to overcome a host of professional and bureaucratic barriers that arise whenever changes are proposed. Some of these barriers are as follows:[4]

1. Professional boundaries and jealousies. Different training and orientation of professions complicate communication (use of different terminology); inhibit teamwork (lack of knowledge of what different fields have to offer and lack of experience in working as a team); threaten job security, control, or individual job satisfaction; and cause the program to be planned without the input of a discipline charged with carrying out the program.

2. Inadequate planning. Program tailored to personal rather than to expressed need; personnel unable to evaluate components of program; program does not meet total health needs.

3. Consumer. Lack of information in community about program; cultural differences; education of parents regarding responsibility for self-care; stereotypes of school health professionals; different expectations, beliefs, life styles, and educational and economic backgrounds; and different degrees of desire to be involved in planning, development, implementation and financing, and rewards for being healthy.

4. Legal. Concerns about malpractice.

5. Finances. Uninformed decision makers (school boards and administrators); lack of long-range commitment.

6. Manpower training. Inability to train sufficient manpower.

7. Politics. Changing local, state, and national priorities; changing composition of school board and personnel; lack of cooperation with private practicing health professionals.

8. Access to services. Inadequate transportation; telephone access; hours of service; appointment systems; emergency care.

9. Support systems. Lack of outreach and community education, nutrition counseling and services, environmental education and services, genetic counseling, social and mental health counseling, home health care, homemaker services, and referral for nonmedical problems.

10. Focus on sickness. Lack of health education and cultural awareness training; focus on physical health.

Planning for Change

Perhaps the element that is most often forgotten in planning programs is change. Programs must be flexible enough to accommodate changes, particularly in funding and personnel. Indeed, the program itself will create change and often require that modifications be made in the goals and objectives. Furthermore, an identical program in two communities might evolve quite differently over time. Social change has a continual effect on people and programs. Such changes are almost impossible to predict, so programs must be organized with this in mind. The change agents and planners who helped evolve the initial school health plan may move, requiring a new organization and new personnel to direct the program. Replacements seldom like to keep things in the same way as their predecessors, but if the program has an effective evaluation mechanism, it is less likely that programs that have been shown to be effective and successful will be terminated by new administrators.

Although we have stressed the individuality of communities in planning school health programs, five general objectives are probably appropriate to most school health programs. In discussing these objectives, examples are given regarding how each objective can be approached. All examples are not necessarily appropriate to all schools.

Objective: Provide Ways to Enhance the Health and Learning Environment of Students

Activities to meet this objective include protection against disease and disability, identification of health problems, and rehabilitation of students with permanent disabilities. Protection against disease and disability during school-supervised activities includes provision of adequate emergency care, evaluation of the health impact of school programs, and prevention of spread of disease within a school.

Example: Provision of Adequate Emergency Care

This activity is elaborated in detail to remind those planning or reviewing health programs that any component, though it might seem simple, requires the time and attention of a number of competent individuals to become operational. There are many steps to assure each student adequate emergency care.

First-aid policies and emergency management instructions that are authoritative and conform to accepted first-aid practices must be provided in a written form that can be used easily by all school staff, adapted to include frequent school accidents (such as knocked out teeth), distributed to all areas where needed, known to school staff, and reviewed periodically to be kept current. A school staff member must be designated to provide first-aid and emergency management on a daily basis. This person must be adequately trained, understand responsibilities, and be available during times the school is responsible for its students. Arrangements must be made for first-aid and emergency care instruction to appropriate staff.

A procedure must be developed to be followed in case of a severe, life-threatening emergency. This should be determined for each school, outlined clearly in writing, and known to the total school staff. The specific responsibility of each participant must be designated, and prior arrangements with local health care providers should be included in instructions. This procedure can be especially valuable in situations outside usual school settings, such as outdoor education camps or in activities with students whose physical condition makes them especially vulnerable to accidents, such as those who have difficulty swallowing because of organic impairment.

Means must be provided for collecting information from each student's parent, including address and telephone numbers where parents can be reached, choice of source of medical care, name of adult whose judgment would be accepted if parent cannot be reached, name of adult who could provide transportation for student, medical condition of student which might make special management necessary (diabetes, blood disease, severe allergy, heart disease, and so on). A system must be developed for keeping this information as current as possible by yearly collection and by requests that schools be notified of any change during the year. Information provided by parents should be filed so it is readily available in case of need. This should include a method of alerting personnel to the presence of a hazardous medical condition in a student.

Also needed is a system for keeping a record of accidents and environment at time of any accident, so conditions can be analyzed with a view toward prevention.

A number of staff members should be involved in reviewing or planning the provision of emergency care. A district level administrator should direct and participate in development of forms and procedures, orient district personnel to the plans, and make possible the provision of necessary personnel, forms, and supplies. This person should decide who is to provide direct first-aid (nurse, health aide, volunteer, or secretary), under whose supervision they will function, and the training to be required. Some districts employ health aides; some use volunteers. The Red Cross sponsors a school health aide program and shares responsibility for training the volunteers. In a few districts, the job description of the school secretary lists as a duty the provision of minor first-aid to students and, as a requirement for continuing employment, yearly attendance at a district-sponsored refresher course.

The administrator of each school should participate in planning, adapt the district plan to his building, orient building staff to the program and the part each is to take, have the recommended supplies and equipment available, and make arrangements for collection of information about students and for its storage and use. The school physician should prepare and recommend first-aid and emergency care procedures, recommend supplies and equipment needed, participate in developing forms and plans for use of information, help make the necessary arrangements for agreements in the community, and participate in orientation or in-service education for staff. The supervisor of school nurses should participate in all aspects of general planning. Additional activities would depend on specific responsibilities assigned to the school nurse. The health educator should participate in all aspects of general planning to incorporate educational aspects with services.

A secretary is needed to do recording, typing, and duplicating. The jobs to be done for continuing operation of program include performing first-aid and emergency care services, periodic review of instructions and forms, orientation and instruction of new personnel expected to administer first-aid, ordering of supplies (this may be done on a district basis from a list of recommended supplies, and requests for supplies requiring special skill such as inflatable splints should be cleared with the person responsible for first-aid instructions), distribution of replacement supplies and materials, periodic replacement of forms, periodic collection and appropriate filing of information necessary for each student, and regular review of daily record of students reporting accidents or illnesses as a method of locating students or situations that need attention.

Review of activities, plans, and programs to evaluate possible effect on health of students can help prevent accidents. Activities planned for a student should be consistent with the student's developmental level. For example, a kindergarten child should not be expected to sit for long periods of time. A junior high student should be provided with adult supervision to stop an activity when the activity becomes hazardous as the student's tiredness increases.

An activity planned outside the school should be reviewed to see that students are adequately prepared and equipped to protect themselves. For example, preparation for an education camp-out should include instructions regarding proper clothing to keep warm, protection against sunburn, or protection from insects— whatever is appropriate for the particular time and place. If a swimming pool is part of the equipment of a school, arrangements should be made to keep any student from being unsupervised in the pool area.

Special arrangements should be made when a student with a health impairment is to participate in a program that would make special planning advisable. For example, if a student with diabetes is to engage in a rigorous schedule of physical activity, his parents should be alerted so either his diet or insulin can be adjusted.

This kind of guidance requires that the school staff have some knowledge of normal growth and development and of possibly hazardous situations for students with disease conditions. Ways to maintain or augment staff knowledge in these areas are discussed later.

Review of new activities, plans, programs to evaluate the possible effects on the health of students, and safeguards that might be included in plans requires a mechanism within the district whereby proposals for new activities are presented to a representative group for consideration. This group should include representatives from administration and from health education, psychology, nursing, and medical services. Such programs as expansion of competitive sports for girls, early entrance to kindergarten, and trampoline use at the intermediate school level deserve consideration.

In attempting to keep students and staff free from communicable disease, several important activities should be considered. Hygienic measures should be taught and followed. Individual protection should be afforded whenever possible.

Example: Prevent Spread of Disease Within School by Exclusion of Sick Individuals

Ill students must be excluded from school. A guide for determining which students should be kept out of school should contain a listing of signs, symptoms, and history indicating possible communicable disease. A procedure for dismissing students from school should include a method for notification of parent, plan for recommendation to parent, and for helping parent find medical care, if necessary.

Ill staff should be excluded from school. Periodic reminders to school staff about good public health procedures to prevent transmission of disease can help. Any screening procedures (for example, tuberculosis screening) required of staff, any unusual disease occurrence (for example, epidemic flu, hepatitis), any unusually stressful occurrence in the school (as in budget cuts with reduction of staff) can be used to disseminate pertinent information as to occurrence, recognition, protection, and sources of help for the condition feared. School staff likely to be alert to above opportunities are those with a strong background in health and illness, such as a health educator, a school nurse, or the school physician.

Example: Prevent Spread of Disease Within a School by Cooperating in Program to Have All Students Immunized According to Local Recommendations

In some states, the type and degree of participation and immunizations required of the school district are designated by law. The steps in instituting an immunization program involve first, planning by the school district, local public health authority, health care providers, and parents to decide the objectives (such as which students are to be immunized, to what disease, what percentage of conformity is acceptable), the responsibilities of each agency or organization (who will pay for biologicals, forms, personnel; who will plan forms, releases, and consents; who will administer immunizations; who will furnish personnel; who will make decisions with possible legal implications; who will keep records of individual students, and what will be kept), the scheduling of activities, and a method for continuing interrelationships and coordination between organizations.

Planning by the school district of details of activities accepted for the district is the second step. This will include the development of a system for notifying parents of requirements for recommendations, the development of procedures for screening students to discover who needs immunizations, and deciding type of record to be kept of an individual student's immunizations. In addition, it will involve preparation of necessary forms and procedures for distribution and collection and disposition of forms. A procedure must be developed for cooperation with other agencies and individuals, and an appropriate school staff member designated to have responsibility in each area above and for district coordination of program. Personnel to be involved from the school district and the time necessary for the activity depends to some extent on how much is required by law and how much has been decided by local option.

Identification of Health Problems and Efforts Toward Remediation Include Screening and Referral Activities

In deciding whether a screening procedure is to be incorporated into the program in any district, certain questions must be considered: Is the procedure required by law? Are there any characteristics of the students of the district that make them particularly vulnerable to the defect the screening procedure is expected to indicate? (Sometimes local health care providers can indicate a high incidence of a specific condition.) Is the present staff able to add this duty without dropping other activities? If not, which is more important, or is there a possibility of adding more staff? If the screening procedure identifies certain students, can remediation or improvement be provided by school staff, or does it require referral to an outside resource? If to an outside resource, is this available? Can the total plan of screening, referring, helping, curing, and using information to improve the student's school program be implemented?[5]

It might be worthwhile to consider whether to institute a particular screening procedure or to conduct an educational campaign so parents, students, and teachers would be more aware of the possibility of the occurrence of a particular defect, which is an informal type of screening in itself. For example, in a community where most students are receiving private medical supervision on a regular basis, is it more valuable to use available staff to teach the possible occurrence, natural history, and expected management of a particular disease? Or is it more valuable to organize and conduct a screening program for the disease in the schools of the area? If the condition being considered affects a large number of students of the community, an educational approach might be preferred. If the condition affects fewer students and general education would not be pertinent, if it is serious for those affected, if it is fairly easy to detect and is treatable, a school screening program might be the best choice. Several types of screening activities are appropriate in the school health setting.

Example: Observational Health Appraisal

School personnel, particularly teachers, have the opportunity to observe deviation by a student from either his own former attitude, performance, or behavior, or from the normal range for his age and developmental group. This type of screening requires that the teacher have adequate knowledge of a student as well as of the usual expectations for the developmental group. Teachers can increase or maintain their observational skills for detecting possible medical defects by attending workshops on topics dealing with what to look for, significance of observations, and what to do with the observations.

A necessary component in obtaining the greatest value from teachers' observations is proper procedure in dealing with the information. In referring after this type of screening, the most helpful information for use in school planning is likely to result if parents are involved early, an outside agency or individual already working with the student or family is seen as concerned with the total situation and as a valuable contributor, parents' wishes regarding source of care are honored and competence of source is assumed, means of adequate written communication between school and source of medical care are provided, and systematic use is made of information received from any medical resource in school management or planning. Health-oriented school staff can use the opportunity afforded by special events at school to alert teachers to observational possibilities. The school district can help the teachers by providing consultation to them from the school nurse, health educator, and school physician. Observational health appraisal might be extended to include students and their parents. In this case, the school can participate by helping students to understand more about illness behavior, the signs and symptoms of disease, and some objective measures of detection of disease, such as taking temperatures. Parents might be assisted by having information about observation of their children and the possible significance of these findings furnished to them at appropriate times.

Example: Vision Screening

In some states, procedures and requirements have been incorporated in laws that are binding on the schools. If this is not so, decisions must be made as to elements of vision to be considered and the screening technique to be used, the population to be screened, whether parental permission is necessary, the personnel to be responsible for the program, and the training and supervision of persons conducting screening. The procedure to be followed in notification to parents of results and referral for further evaluation must be designed as well as the records to be kept and the preparation and content of work forms and referral sheets. Joint planning involving administration, school nurse, school physician, and appropriate community groups is important.

Example: Screening Programs

Vision and hearing screening traditionally have been seen as a potential for uncovering defects that would directly affect a student's school performance. In addition, a number of other screening procedures have been carried out in different school districts. General steps for implementation are similar to those for vision screening. Some of these are screening by record evaluation and screening for scoliosis, poor growth, diabetes, abnormal blood pressure, dental disease, and voice defects.

Preventing Further Complications in a Student with a Handicap Which Is Not Totally Remediable Is a Concern of the School

Staff awareness of recommended management and educational implications of certain medical conditions will often augment medical treatment and help prevent the development of a further handicap. Proper classroom management of a student with an orthopedic defect can add hours of benefit from a treatment standpoint and prevent increasing deformity. Understanding of a chronic condition can result in school management of the situation which helps prevent added psychological problems for a student (as in asthma or epilepsy).

The increasing awareness of students regarding ways to live with their medical conditions should lead to a fuller life. The school may take the initiative in planning, after consultation with a student's health care provider, to help the student understand more about himself and his total situation and what this means in terms of adjustment to school. For example, a student who is required to take stimulant medication, and needs to be taught by a special instructional method, can adjust better if his fears are allayed that something more serious or progressive is present. He will have a better basis on which to plan his future life and career if he understands the total situation. One example of a program to support and rehabilitate students is the Health Education Learning Program (HELP) for students with asthma. As a group, students with asthma share special educational needs. They must learn to cope with this chronic illness as well as with the demands of school and other daily activities. HELP is a cooperative school health education program involving physicians, nurses, teachers, counselors, and social workers to assist students and parents in developing personal skills in the management of asthma.[6]

Objective: Provide a Bridge Between School Health Services and Health Care Providers in the Community

Best communication is possible if persons trying to communicate have mutual respect for and understanding of one another. Planned efforts toward this situation usually are necessary.

Example:

Scheduled no-host luncheon meetings, held on a regular basis, are a helpful activity that any interested health care provider and any interested school staff member can attend. This requires only that suitable arrangements be made and that school representation be adequate on all occasions, including educators and administrators as well as special services personnel.

Example:

If the school physician maintains membership in local medical groups and on local hospital staffs and keeps alert to appropriate opportunities to explain programs of the schools, assistance and cooperation of health care providers will be enhanced.

Example:

In addition, school health workshops or meetings planned jointly by the school district and health care providers are of benefit to all aspects of the program. Each group must consider routinely the contributions and prerogatives of the other in dealing with students about whom both are concerned.

Example:

Including representatives of health care providers in decision-making groups will help when decisions affect the health and welfare of the providers' patients (planning special programs, procedures, and so on).

Example:

Health care providers can be supplied with information regarding any new services or activities of medical significance within the school district. For instance, at the time new procedures were instituted as the result of the national Family Rights and Privacy Act,[7] health care providers in some districts were notified of these changes. Regular, periodic communications regarding students should occur between providers and school personnel. School entrance reports from physicians, notification of placement of child after contributing information from physician has been received, specific requests from physicians to be carried out at school, report of progress if a student has a chronic, continuing problem or if a student is receiving maintenance medication serve such a purpose. These interactions are accomplished fairly simply if proper forms are prepared and the responsibility for such communication is assigned to a specific member of the school staff.

Referral: To Provide a Bridge Between School Health Services and Health Care Providers in the Community

In reviewing or establishing such a procedure a number of activities are needed. First is to decide the reasons a student is to be referred. This might be clearance for physical activity or for a special school program, or because the signs or symptoms of a possible pathologic condition have been observed and medical evaluation or treatment is desired.

A decision needs to be made whether referrals are to be made routinely to a general physician or for specialist care. The coordinating function of the general physician is important in the continuing medical supervision of the student. What information is to be requested from the physician must be decided. Are all referrals to be written, and if not, which are?

Forms for written communication based on the above decisions need to be prepared. The person to initiate referral must be determined, as well as how information is to be routed and who is to receive the reply. This should be written out as a procedure. Consent forms need to be developed to conform to the Family Rights and Privacy Act. Instruction of school staff regarding procedures must be arranged, and a procedure for appropriate school personnel to be made aware of information returned to school needs to be established.

Objective: Assist Students and Their Parents To Become More Responsible and Assertive About Their Own Health

One approach to this objective is through sharing responsibilities with the home. A delicate distinction needs to be made between sharing and usurping the responsibility and prerogatives of the family of a child attending school. Observations of a child in the school setting and in group activity, and judging changes in his appearance, performance, and behavior or significant differences from his peers can be done well by trained school personnel. Supplying parents with information about concerns resulting from these observations is expected of school personnel. The decision as to the future course to be followed in evaluation and, if possible, remediation for a problem, is one in which the school can have a vital influence; but ultimately it is made by the parent. A positive approach from school personnel includes recognition that most parents are eager to help their children, that expectations of the family might be different from that of the school, that parents may not be aware of resources from which they can obtain help or of how to request care, and that parents might be reluctant to use available resources. In all these areas, which lead to the final decision of the parent, school personnel can take an active, supportive part.

Example: Use of Home-School Agent

In the Galveston, Texas, public schools, the home-school agents, who are community persons with special qualifications, are accepted by the families with whom they work (see Chapter 3). Following a specific training program given by the district, the home-school agent assists students to get adequate medical care and families to assume responsibility for obtaining care.

The school program can build or foster communications between the home, the school, and the health care system. School personnel communicating with parents of students who have health problems can provide help for these students and their families in identifying ongoing sources of health care by home visit, by telephone, by letter, or by form.

Example:

Regular, periodic communication with parents regarding the health of students will strengthen the contacts and interactions. The kindergarten entrance history, yearly emergency information, notification to parent of an occurrence in school, and notification regarding advisability of immunization booster are among the helpful communications that school personnel can initiate.

Example:

A file or directory of community health resources made available to students and their families is of benefit.

Example:

Holding a "health fair" in a school or school district can bring together students, parents, school personnel, health care providers, and other interested community members.

The development of health education programs that teach necessary individual skills is a third activity to help students and parents toward being more responsible for their own health. Good health education is a necessary part of a school health program. Health education can involve instruction, special projects, modeling, or group activities. In planning health curricula, there are many opportunities to integrate health instruction with other activities in the schools.

An effective health education program should focus on behavioral outcomes rather than just giving information, and it must deal with developing skills in making decisions for which the decision maker is responsible. To develop interest, the program must be at the student's level of understanding and be pertinent to his interests. Techniques of presentation, methods, materials, and equipment must be available to the teachers, and the teachers must either know or be assisted in how to proceed.

Example:

HELP for students with asthma, described previously, is a prime example. Preparing a description of existing health education activities and assessing the receptivity of a school district and a community to specific ideas of health education provide a helpful background preliminary to planning or enlarging a health education program. Inclusion of health-oriented school staff in considering the curriculum is valuable.

Planned participation by health-oriented staff members in classroom activities can be useful to enhance instruction by the teacher. Community education programs might be offered by the school staff on many subjects, including diet, nutrition, and stretching a budget. Learning programs can be developed for students with special health problems, as well as programs expected to develop skills in health-related behavior.

Objective: Utilize Educational and Health Manpower Resources Effectively and Efficiently in Enhancing the Health and Learning Environment of Students

Use of health personnel by the school should be determined according to needs of students, to resources in the community, to the philosophy of health services in the district, and to objectives accepted for district health programs.

Health personnel can be used in different ways: in teaming, in consultation, and for provision of direct services. To improve the program, at times it might be advisable to plan health-oriented training for certain members of school or district staff.

For teaming to work, individuals from different disciplines must be available on the district staff. Representatives from each discipline must recognize their own specific and particular contribution but also be aware of areas where competencies of different disciplines overlap. Each individual and each discipline must respect the other members of the team and work cooperatively. When understanding and appreciation among team members is not sufficient, a plan should be made by the responsible administrators to foster this understanding.

To accomplish teaming within a school, a plan must be devised whereby all members of the team are alerted when there is a concern about a student. All should have access to all information available about that student. The best service is provided when each discipline is allowed to decide whether it has something to offer.

A possible administrative arrangement is a procedure in which each student who is of special concern to a staff member (usually the teacher) is made known to the principal or his designee. Each team member reviews and evaluates the situation from the viewpoint of his discipline and suggests further steps in evaluation or remediation, and a mechanism is provided for correlation of information from team members. Another possibility is a regularly scheduled team meeting to allow the same activities to be accomplished.

With either system, the primary health care provider should be included when consideration is being given to a student under his care. A team leader needs to be designated so all participants know who is to make a final decision in case of conflict, who is to schedule meetings when necessary, who is to be responsible for coordinating the plan decided by team, how advice generated through the team is to be put into use by the teacher, and what kind of records are to be kept and where.

To accomplish teaming on a district level, the representatives of all disciplines need to have regular, informational communication regarding activities of all disciplines. An opportunity to participate in district planning should be given to representatives when activities that involve their disciplines are considered or discussed. Also, persons from each discipline should have an opportunity to suggest to school administrators their areas of possible contribution.

Health personnel can be used also through consultation. Effective consultation depends on mutual respect and understanding between the persons requesting and those providing consultation. It is necessary that each participant be competent in his own field, that the consultation be requested, not imposed, and that each participant have a clear idea of what is expected.

Because of limitations of time and money, it may be necessary to plan for only some of the services that a consultant could offer. When this occurs, it is likely that a negotiated decision between those requesting consultation and the person undertaking to provide consultation will result in the best service and greatest help.

The need for consultation will be determined by the definition of the school health program adopted by the school district. Since physician consultation might be expected in any school health program, medical consultation is the most ready example to elaborate. Similar points should be considered, however, when consultation from any other disciplinary field is to be arranged.

Example: Medical Consultation

"For future planning of school health programs, a distinction must be made between 'medicine in the school' and 'school medicine.' 'School medicine' is an area of medical practice concerned with the identification, observation, and management of health problems in the school setting. It has its own body of knowledge and skills and is not a part of medical practice in which all physicians are competent automatically because of their basic medical education and experience."[8]

For most effective service, it is necessary that school physicians be placed administratively so they can be included in the formulation of school district policies or procedures concerned with the health and safety of students and school personnel. They should have access to the superintendent, heads of other divisions or sections, and principals. School physicians should be available to personnel of the school district who have questions relating to medical facts, procedures, policies, and ethics.

To provide the best service, the physician must have the opportunity to participate in policy making and program planning in many areas, including physical education, competitive athletics, management of students presenting symptoms of possibly correctable physical or emotional problems, management of students with permanent handicaps that interfere with full participation in the school program, health education, communicable disease control, first-aid, and emergency care. Since physicians can contribute to many aspects of the school program, they should be allowed this flexibility instead of being placed in only one service, for example health services or guidance services.

Certain suggestions can be made to arrange for the school physician to have an opportunity to learn more about the total school program and to develop ideas as to how medicine might contribute. The physician could be included on the list to which agenda or minutes of most meetings in the district are sent. These could include such groups as the school board, the superintendent's cabinet, the principals, the total administrative group, curriculum commission, nursing staff, and guidance and counseling staff. Second, the physician should be included on the mailing list of any informative material sent to parents from either central administrative or local school sources. In addition, the physician can be included on the list to receive any communication sent from the school staff regarding community health care individuals or agencies.

As to qualifications, school physicians should have an interest in children and young people and training or experience in working with them. They should know the scientific basis and techniques of various school health screening tests and examinations, the general provisions of laws and regulations governing school health, and the functions of other school personnel, such as psychologists, guidance counselors, special teachers. He should be able to assist with identification and appropriate management of school-related emotional and learning problems. Also, he needs to be aware of standards for the school physical environment, desirable employee health practices and programs, organization of emergency plans, and safe athletic practices and equipment. An important area with which he should be familiar is the legal and administrative structure of the school district in which he works.[9]

In addition to participation in teaming activities and for consultation, health personnel may provide direct services to children.

Example: Provision of Direct Services

One school district and their local health care providers have agreed that treatment for head lice can be recommended by school personnel under standing orders from the school physician. Head lice are common among students in some schools; and, since it is often difficult and costly to obtain treatment, requiring that the whole family be involved, standing orders facilitate the provision of care for this condition.

Training programs for school staff might be needed to develop new competencies. Each person on the school staff has skills and knowledge as a result of his background, training, and experience. Although each of the professionally trained individuals has certain areas that are peculiar to the training of his particular discipline, a number of areas of competence are found within more than one discipline. Also, undeveloped competencies are often found in some disciplines that can be enhanced by individuals from another profession.

Many teachers and other school staff with no formal medical training can be helped to become astute observers for reactions of students indicating a possible medical problem. To increase this competency, districts can help by providing funds for substitutes or released time for staff to attend in-service programs, credit courses, workshops, or meetings. Districts can plan and sponsor workshops within their jurisdiction. Appropriate topics for such formal training sessions are "medical aspects of learning problems," "observation of students," "child growth and development," and "emergencies in the school." Districts can also participate in field training of students from teacher-training institutions, making sure that the health-oriented staff of the district have a chance to contribute to the training of the student teacher.

Increased competence and understanding of health-oriented professions in the area of schools and education and in the part played in health of students also can be fostered by cooperating with professional schools to provide experiences for students from the health professions.

Health-oriented staff in the school can contribute in an informal way to the ability of other staff to increase their confidence in evaluating health of students by attending regular staff and faculty meetings, observing needs, and being alert to opportunities to increase knowledge of staff about students and their health needs, sources of help, and how to obtain desired help.

Objective: Periodically Assess the Outcomes of Health Services Provided in the School and in the Community

How Well Have We Done?

Evaluation is a crucial part of any school health program. It should be carried out by the program designers as well as by outsiders who have no vested interests in the program or its outcome. The methods used in evaluation and the kinds of information desired should be related to the study purposes.[10] The results of the evaluation, however, should answer questions such as: What are the differences between those who participated in the program versus those who did not? What difference did the program make among the participants; that is, did the program create any changes in the individuals as a result of its intervention? In what ways was the program successful, and in what ways did it fail? What was the cost per unit of output? Can the program be replicated elsewhere; why or why not? What modifications in the program, its objectives, and operation would be suggested as a result of the experience?

The evaluation of a program should measure the degree of effectiveness of each objective. Too often a program's success or failure is assessed by whether it has achieved the overall goal. It is possible for a program to have achieved some objectives and failed to achieve others and still not be considered a total failure. Indeed, one of the purposes of evaluation is to learn the stumbling blocks that occur in working toward achieving certain objectives. The objectives might have been adequate, but the methods of translating them into program activities might have been the reason for not meeting them.

How well a program has succeeded is not to be equated with whether clients are happier now than they were before the program was started. Programs create change whether they are designed to do so or not. Changes that result will not always benefit all parties in the same way or to the same degree. The changes that programs create usually provide the stimulus for or point out the need for additional programs. Thus, the cycle continues. It is often said that the best ideas are those undergoing change. Similarly, school health programs must be constantly susceptible to new ideas and to the changing needs of students, the schools, and the community.

Evaluation covers judgments of many kinds. In essence, evaluation means judging merit. Someone is examining and weighing a phenomenon against some explicit or implicit yardstick. School health programs are usually designed to improve the health of people. The programs are diverse. They can be aimed to change people's knowledge, attitudes, values, behaviors, or the community in which they live. Their common characteristic is the goal of making life better for the people they serve. Programs must be evaluated, therefore, to make the judging process more accurate and objective. Evaluation establishes specific criteria for success. It collects evidence from a representative sample of the units of concern, translates the evidence into qualitative terms, and compares it with the criteria that were set prior to the program. It then draws conclusions about the effectiveness, merit, and success of the program.[11]

Evaluation Questions

The evaluation questions asked most frequently can be grouped into four categories:[12]

1. Appropriateness. These questions are directed toward the importance of the specific problems addressed by the program and their respective relevance or priority. Were the program objectives worthwhile, and do they have a high priority compared with other objectives or programs?
2. Adequacy. Objectives are usually directed toward eliminating a problem that gave rise to the program. Questions concerning how much of the program is directed toward overcoming the problem refers to the adequacy of program objectives.
3. Effectiveness. Programs differ in the extent to which they attain objectives. Given the amount of time, effort, and resources, how successful was the program? Could the program have successfully reached its stated objectives with less time, effort, and resources?
4. Efficiency. Program efficiency is defined as the cost in resources in attaining objectives. Efficiency might be unrelated to appropriateness, adequacy, or effectiveness. Although cost benefit analyses are often viewed as a necessary evil, most granting agencies require that such analyses be included in the evaluation of a program. Though costs vary and change, cost analyses are rough guides for planning subsequent programs.

When the above four categories of questions are asked about a program, they constitute an evaluation of performance. O.L. Deniston and his colleagues have outlined a model to evaluate program effectiveness.[13] The model is primarily for use by program personnel to evaluate certain aspects of their own performance. However, an outside evaluator can also use it. Regardless of who performs the evaluation, it should be remembered that the purpose of evaluation is improvement. Therefore, program evaluation should be endorsed by those who have the authority to make changes.

The Deniston model does not offer a systematic procedure for assessing the impact of unplanned activities. All programs have side effects. Indeed, the proof of program effectiveness or ineffectiveness is often found in the way program activities were conducted. Evaluation efforts, therefore, should include some assessment of process.

School Health: The Proof Is in the Process

School health programs are usually continued or discontinued on the outcome of the evaluation of the program; that is, whether the program achieved its objectives. *How* and *why* the objectives were or were not met are often overlooked in the evaluative process. The objectives represent one point in the process of school health. The long, involved process of achieving teamwork among disciplines and between disciplines and parents and between all of these and administrators and politicians often tells more about what can be achieved with respect to school health in a given community. Process is not easily quantifiable, so its documentation in anecdotal form may be viewed as "soft" and "unconvincing" to hard-line decision makers. Yet, *how* school health programs succeed or fail often is the key to understanding why success or failure occurred. Indeed, all parties involved in planning, implementing, and participating in school health programs should themselves be changed in some way as a result of doing school health.

A Guide for Doing School Health

In an attempt to present a practical outline of the activities that would help achieve a successful school health program, we have summarized in Table 4-1 the major objectives of a school health program and some of the ways to reach the objectives listed. This table can be used as a reference for school administrators and others in assessing how far they have traveled at any point along the continuum from planning to practice, if they accept the objectives in Table 4-1 as their objectives.

Table 4-1 Objectives of a School Health Program and Steps Toward Achieving Them

Provide Ways to Enhance the Health and Learning Environment of Students	Provide a Bridge Between School Health Services and Health Care Providers in the Community	Assist Students and Their Parents to Become More Responsible and Assertive About Their Own Health	Utilize Educational and Health Manpower Resources Effectively and Efficiently in Enchancing the Health and Learning Environment of Students	Periodically Assess the Outcomes of Health Services Provided in the School and in the Community

A. Assure adequate emergency care
 	
B. Prevent spread of disease within school
  1. Exclude ill students and staff from school
  2. Initiate or cooperate in immunization program(s)
 	
C. Screening. Evaluate proposed screening procedures (observational health appraisal, vision screening, learning screening, others) by the following criteria:
  1. Is it required by law?
  2. Are local students especially vulnerable?
  3. Can present staff perform this duty without dropping others? Or can more staff be added?
	A. Maintain and develop understanding and respect between involved groups by considering the contributions and prerogatives of others
	
	B. Provide effective referral procedures
	  1. Identify reasons student is to be referred
	  2. Decide whether referrals to general physician are to be routine
	  3. Decide what information is to be requested
	  4. Decide which referrals are to be written (are all?)
	  5. Prepare forms for written communication
	  6. Decide who is to initiate procedure, how to route, who to receive information
		A. Sharing responsibilities with the home
		
		B. Utilizing or developing communications between home-school-health care systems
		  1. School health personnel offer information on health care resources to families of identified student—by visit, phone, letter, or form
		
		C. Develop educational programs
		  1. Health-oriented staff participate on a planned basis in classroom activities
		  2. Develop community education programs
		  3. Develop learning programs for students with special health problems
			A. Teaming within the school and within the district
			
			B. Consultation—cooperation needs to be arranged with competent experts
			
			C. Provision of direct services
			
			D. Training programs and workshops
				A. Evaluation included in all plans
				
				B. Benefits to students are criteria

Table 4-1 (Continued)

Provide Ways to Enhance the Health and Learning Environment of Students	Provide a Bridge Between School Health Services and Health Care Providers in the Community	Assist Students and Their Parents to Become More Responsible and Assertive About Their Own Health	Utilize Educational and Health Manpower Resources Effectively and Efficiently in Enchancing the Health and Learning Environment of Students	Periodically Assess the Outcomes of Health Services Provided in the School and in the Community
4. Can any remedy or improvement be offered by staff to students identified, or is an outside source available? 5. Can the total plan be put into effect? D. Prevent complications—rehabilitation	7. Develop consent forms 8. Arrange for instruction of school staff on procedures 9. Arrange for appropriate school personnel to receive information returned			

REFERENCES

1. R. J. Haggerty, "Child Health: Options for the Community and the Schools," keynote address, National School Health Conference, Galveston, Texas, June 21, 1976.

2. G.L. McAndrew, "Changing Systems to Meet Child Health Needs: The Gary Story," presented at National School Health Conference, Galveston, Texas, June 22, 1976.

3. H. B. Long, R. C. Anderson, and J. A. Blubaugh, Eds., *Approaches to Community Development* (Iowa City: National University Extension Association and The American College Testing Program, 1973).

4. "Doctors and Dollars Are Not Enough: How to Improve Health Services for Children and Their Families," A Report by the Children's Defense Fund of the Washington Research Project, Inc. (Washington, D.C.: April 1976), Publisher: Children's Defense Fund.

5. W.K. Frankenburg and B.W. Camp, Eds., *Pediatric Screening Tests* (Springfield, Ill.: Charles C. Thomas, 1975).

6. G. S. Parcel and P. R. Nader, "Evaluation of a Pilot School Health Education Program for Asthmatic Children," *Journal of School Health* 47, no. 8 (Oct. 1977): 453.

7. P.L. 93-38, The Protection of the Rights and Privacy of Parents and Students, August 30, 1974.

8. Committee on School Health, American Academy of Pediatrics, *School Health: A Guide for Physicians* (1972), p. 23.

9. E. Bryan *et al.*, "The School Physician in Special Education," *Journal of School Health* 47, no. 8 (Oct. 1977): 486.

10. "Preventive Medicine USA: Theory, Practice and Application of Prevention in Personal Health Services," Task Force Report sponsored by John E. Fogarty International Center and American College of Preventive Medicine (New York: Prodist, 1976).

11. C. H. Weiss, *Evaluation Research: Methods of Assessing Program Effectiveness* (Englewood Cliffs, N.J.: Prentice-Hall, 1972).

12. O. L. Deniston, I. M. Rosenstock, and V. A. Getting, "Evaluation of Program Effectiveness," in H. C. Schulberg, A. Sheldon, and F. Baker, Eds., *Program Evaluation in the Health Fields* (New York: Behavioral Publications, 1969).

13. *Ibid.*

Chapter 5

Community Studies at the National School Health Conference: An Exercise in Options for School Health

James Williams, M.S.W.
and Susan Gilman, M.S.

When the National School Health Conference convened in Galveston in June 1976, the participants arrived full of enthusiasm and high expectations. The ideas and concepts that had been communicated in the pre-conference announcements and materials had aroused a wave of interest far more intense than anyone could have anticipated.*

What happened at the conference (principally in the unique Community Study sessions), what have been the intensely interesting experiences of these communities in the years that followed, and how the enthusiasm of the conference participants was sustained while their expectations took several new directions form the subject matter of this chapter.

ROLE OF COMMUNITY STUDIES

The outstanding events of the National School Health Conference, according to the participants' evaluation, were the Community Study sessions. Several selected communities and cities in Texas (and, serendipitously, Massachusetts) were invited to send teams to the conference that were composed of key persons representing the health care industry, the educational system, and the community itself. These teams were to be "living" case studies, presenting the current state of school health in their respective communities. The Community Study sessions were the

---

*For a detailed accounting of the preparation and process of the National School Health Conference, see the Appendix.

forums that tested the validity of the objectives and methods that we were trying to develop against the concrete experiences of the subject communities. All who attended the conference had the opportunity to participate in one of the problem-solving case studies.

It should be understood that this chapter is in no way intended as a scientific study. The outcomes described represent the judgments and interpretation of those who put the conference together. The description of the communities that follows summarizes individual responses from evaluation forms at the conference, preliminary results from a one-year follow-up survey, and numerous informal contacts and interviews with participants in the communities under examination. Our assessments are necessarily incomplete; but we have found them to be instructive, provocative, and stimulating—leading to some thoughts and observations that we feel could have significance in the future of school health. The important point to remember is that the whole group was responsible for producing the outcomes. Whatever resulted from the Community Study sessions depended on the participation of everyone present.

Attempting to do justice to the efforts of the four community teams presents several problems. Just as their experiences have been different since the conference, the levels of available information about those experiences varies from one to another. The approach at the conference of using many facilitators, although useful for many reasons, created difficulties in consistent recordkeeping. Information on how groups worked is difficult to preserve; at best, it is very perishable. In addition to the recording at the conference and the informative discussions at that time, data sources for this chapter include a follow-up survey sent to all conference participants, occasional personal contacts with some participants, contacts with others who are familiar with activities in these communities, and limited telephone interviews conducted after the survey.

The descriptions of the four communities that follow are the authors' interpretation of the available information.* These vignettes are not comparisons; they are an effort to capture some of the significance of a series of important events in the life of each school and community. It is hoped that members of these communities will forgive any distortions and will be sympathetic with this effort to be faithful to their intentions.

COMMUNITY STUDY: ODESSA, TEXAS

The Odessa story lends itself well to analysis. The community team came to Galveston for the conference with the expressed purpose of

---

* All data quoted in this chapter with reference to the individual communities are taken from the community profile materials prepared by each community team for the presentation or from notes of discussions following those presentations.

developing a model school health program for a school system and community such as theirs. With the resources of the community, as well as the possibility of cooperation by the school administration and the board of education, such a model could be forthcoming in the near future.

There is something to be said for the prevailing optimism one finds, particularly, in many parts of Texas and in the southwest generally. "Can't" is not a word one often hears. Much about Odessa expresses that spirit.

The steering committee selected the school system in Odessa as a potential community study for several reasons. The city and its schools seemed to be of such a size, with an adequate balance between needs and resources, that real possibilities existed to develop the type of comprehensive school health program toward which the conference aimed. The existing pattern of school health in the schools was a familiar one, with many health and education services performed for students by school nurses and other personnel, but with the whole system organized into traditional vertical structures and little formal interaction or communication taking place between the major divisions.

Odessa is a vigorous small city of approximately 110,000, located in the vast oil-rich Permian Basin of west Texas. It is small enough for personal interaction between the leadership of the schools and city and its citizens, yet large enough to support an adequate range of health and human resources. Employment statistics are consistently excellent when compared with the nation; and although petroleum-related industries are the base for the economy, sufficient diversification is present to ensure continued stability.

Certainly every city has its problems, and Odessa is no exception, But the relatively low incidence of urban problems usually experienced by a city Odessa's size makes it an unusual place. The schools are modern and well regarded throughout the state and have avoided most typical problems in obtaining resources. Adequate schools and educational programs for the children of Odessa are a community priority.

When initial contact was made with the schools to explore the possibility of Odessa's becoming a Community Study, the response was immediate and positive. A meeting was set up in the office of the superintendent to include key people in the administration involved with education and health, as well as some community leaders. Several conference steering committee members traveled to Odessa. After several hours of discussion, the decision was made to participate.

At this point a team was formed to prepare for the conference, and the chairman of the conference steering committee was designated as the liaison person for the team. During the three months that followed, the team met regularly, assessed their school health activities, and finally decided on a problem on which to work at the conference. An attractive community profile package and slide show was prepared. The liaison person made several visits to meet with the team and assist in their preparation.

During this period the team struggled to define a problem on which to concentrate, as outlined in the guidelines (see the Appendix). Although everyone could identify some areas where they could do better, there seemed to be no outstanding issues that fit the description of a "problem." It finally occurred to the team that no organizational structure existed to work on any of the problems within the scope of school health—the team members who worked in narrow areas of the schools' adminstration had no mechanism to work *together* to solve the problems in school health and to develop a comprehensive program. Planning had been essentially incremental; links between services and education were not adequate. In all this, the group was presenting almost a textbook case of current school health programs and their vicissitudes. Out of their work came the statement of the problem they brought to the conference: *How can we in Odessa, Texas, plan, coordinate, and administer a better and more comprehensive school health program than now exists?*

The Odessa team presented a well-prepared program at the Community Study session. The participants were lively and the interaction brisk. The Odessa team willingly received assistance in focusing their objectives in a fashion different from the one presented. They developed a statement of their objective and a series of steps to take upon returning. This session seemed to follow the guideline almost perfectly. After the afternoon workshop, the team met that evening on their own to revise their plan along lines developed in the sessions and were ready for the closing session on the next day.

When the conference concluded, the Odessa team returned home with the following objective and seven steps for action on their problem.

Objective: Develop a plan to evaluate the status of the present health program and define the responsibilities of the school in designing and implementing a comprehensive health program for students.

Step 1: Write report (including history of group, list of concerns, and people who contributed) back to the superintendent.

Step 2: Appoint/establish a steering committee (developed from Odessa team) and an advisory committee (heterogeneous and broad-based).
Action: To be determined by committee; that is, size, composition, disciplines.

Step 3: Determine existing resources available in the community.

Step 4: State a tentative philosophy: "Education for health rather than health for education."

Step 5: Determine needs—accept constant feedback from the community.
Action: Community survey, possibly done by advisory committee.
Change: Reallocation of resources. Possible change in community attitudes.

Step 6: Appoint professional coordinator of health programs. Coordinator needs to understand education, health, and *children*.
Action: Define the role of the person. Allocate funds.
Change: Some change in organizational structure of school system.

Step 7: Design a program to include ongoing evaluation.

With their Galveston experiences to guide them, the Odessa team continued to meet. A detailed report on the National School Health Conference was presented to the superintendent of schools in July following the conference. A detailed plan was developed from the steps and a proposal presented to the school board the following fall, detailing a seven-step plan and setting up a formal structure for a Steering Committee for School Health. Most significantly, a broad-based advisory committee, composed of people representing many concerns in the community as well as the schools, was formed.

The school board approved the plan and the appointment of the committee. Several subcommittees were formed to work on each step of the plan and met regularly for several months, beginning in January 1977. In the early spring, approximately nine months following the conference, the Steering Committee for School Health recommended an action program to the school district. This program included increasing the health services staff by adding two nurses, aides, clerical people, and a coordinator of health services.

By autumn 1977 the school board had funded two additional nursing positions. The aides' and health services coordinator's positions are yet to be funded, but indications are that they will be picked up as the program develops. Currently an assistant to the coordinator of physical education serves as the health services coordinator.

The steering committee and the advisory committee have remained active and have seen progress in many of the specific problem areas that were identified by the planning and study, including: the development of a referral system, improved communications throughout the schoo system on issues related to health of children, designing of revisions for health curricula for elementary and secondary schools, and improved relationships with the health care system in the community.

The reaction of the conference participants from Odessa to the past year was quite positive. They felt the formation of the advisory committee definitely helped to overcome the lack of knowledge and understanding in the community by providing a means of communication with a variety of people. The broad nature of the committee structure served to legitimize its proposals with the school board. It seems that Odessa is only beginning to realize the potential that lies in involving the community in school health.

COMMUNITY STUDY: AUSTIN, TEXAS

The experience of the Austin community study team is a classic example of the fact that change, whether planned or not, is a fundamental characteristic of social systems. The team came together in preparation for the conference, planned and presented an extensive analysis of the current state of school health in a large urban school district, identified a problem to be attacked that was essential in their newly developing school health program, and then had to watch as events over which they had little or no control determined the outcome of most of their efforts for the past year.

Austin was the largest community to be represented in the Community Study sessions. Located in central Texas, it is considered to be the most attractive city in Texas and consistently turns up on the lists of good places to live in the United States—environmentally, socially, and economically. It is a city, but a manageable one, with a population approaching 300,000 if the students of the University of Texas are included. The state capital and its agencies are located in Austin, as are the county government and the headquarters for the regional planning council. Urban problems do exist, but in numbers and a magnitude that have not overwhelmed the city's resources or morale. Many cities in the country would gladly trade their own problems for some of Austin's, as a large number of these problems are related to the fact that Austin has been one of the fastest growing cities over the past decade. It is considered to be economically stable, with a high percentage of the employment being in white collar positions and "clean" industry. Austin has the reputation of being a moderately liberal community politically, certainly more than Texas in general. The schools are well supported, with a high percentage master's level teachers and a history of sound education and constantly expanding services for children.

The decision to ask Austin school health personnel to prepare a Community Study grew out of the fact that it could represent a major school district in an urban area without being so swamped with complex problems as to make a workshop presentation impracticable.

When the contact was made with the school district, it was positively received because of a recent development in their school health program. For the previous 30 years school nursing services had been provided through a contract with the city-county health department. In 1974 a special study by the school board had recommended that the school system terminate this arrangement and develop its own service for school nurses, and when the school district was approached by the conference steering committee the new health services had been in existence about six months. All the problems of integrating a new service into the existing structure and coordinating it with health education were in the process of being worked on. Administrators felt that the work of preparing a Community Study would be very useful; the steering committee felt that the situation would provide an interesting and challenging Community Study. On this basis, the decision was made to proceed.

The community study team was formed and went to work on its presentation under the guidelines developed by the conference steering committee. The problem on which they decided to work at the conference described exactly where they were in the development of their health services. It was stated as a general question with several components.

How can we in the Austin Independent School District establish and make better use of administration for the promotion of student health?

In a detailed presentation of the problem, the team members presented information on how the problem related to the size of the school system, the present administrative structure, the intermediate structure, and the size of the health services. Specific reference was made to the fact that the health service was new— and different from anything that existed before, that there is a lack of a total systemwide program with integrated services, that role definition for health personnel is an urgent problem, and that health education and health services have a low priority in the Austin Independent School District. It was the last two points—the role definition and the priority level—on which the team desired to focus at the conference.

The presentation to the Community Study session was well prepared, and the problem was discussed at length. Although the problem in all its aspects looked similar to problems faced by school health programs anywhere, the Community Study session participants went to work on it and, with the team, came up with some direction for action. Although the details were worked out on three pages, with many excellent suggestions for strategy to bring about change, the plan actually had four essential elements: institutionalizing of the Austin community team as the planning body for school health, developing a master plan for school health for the district with strategies for implementation, educating the principals and the educational administration on school health and how to use it effectively, and involving the community in school health. Basic to the plan were identifying the kind of organizational structure that would be necessary and developing the strategy to influence the decision makers to adopt the plan.

To examine the results it is necessary to go back to the week before the conference. A long and involved interaction between the Austin Independent School District and the federal court over the form that desegregation would take in Austin finally came to a head during that week. The plan that the court approved required a major readjustment by the school district and many decisions to be made in a short period. Several members of the original Community Study team, including top administrators and school board members interested in school health, had to cancel their trip to Galveston to attend emergency meetings on the crisis in Austin. This set the stage for what was to happen to the proposed plan of action on school health during the coming year. It has not been possible to implement any action toward the development of the master plan due to the priority demands of both time and funds by the desegregation issue. It is ironic that this would happen in a community that is generally seen as being more open on social issues than most.

Individual responses from participants and from others familar with the recent situation in Austin indicate that some gains have been made in school health in specific areas. Many people are working hard to develop the school health service within the constraints of the situation. The integration of the new school nursing roles into the system has moved ahead, though not without some pain and attrition. Several people report numerous individual gains for themselves and their work as a result of the conference. Some report that health education has developed more than expected under the circumstances. Others indicate that schools are beginning to use the health services a little more effectively and that parents are recognizing the usefulness of the new RN roles.

Generally, however, reports are more discouraging than positive, particularly on issues of communication and coordination among services and with the educational administration. Also, priorities have been a source of discouragement. Some personnel who came to Galveston for the conference are no longer with the schools. The new organizational structure that is needed, the "master plan," still does not exist. And, as the priorities of time and funds still seem to be dominated by the desegregation issue, it would appear that the plans and strategies suggested in the Community Study session in 1976 are needed now more than ever before.

It should be noted that this attempt to describe these outcomes for school health in Austin is done with sympathy and understanding; it does not criticize the school administration or the school board. As was stated at the beginning of this section, events in social systems can intersect the best of plans and make it difficult to gain control over the pace or the direction of change.

The school health needs of Austin seem to vindicate the school board's original decision to bring school nursing into the school system. Events since that time powerfully demonstrate that it is not enough to patch in programs and expect to meet the health needs of children. To withstand the pressures of unexpected crisis, as well as to administer a complex array of programs, school health must have a solid *organizational* arrangement. This will make it possible for its essential personnel and programs to maintain their priority and become effective advocates for the health of children.

COMMUNITY STUDY: WORCESTER, MASSACHUSETTS

Worcester, Massachusetts, has become a city committed to school health services. A School Health Council was formed after the National School Health Conference, drawing representatives from the city school and health departments and from the University of Massachusetts Medical School. The council is chaired by a representative of the city manager's office and staffed by a member of the city's human services department. The staff member has a background in human services planning and has facilitated the council's operation by his ability to accomplish the administrative and planning tasks necessary for revamping the program.

To many who were familiar with the situation in Worcester, where the schools and the public health department must interact to provide school health services, the above paragraph must seem astounding. To many participants at the conference who only attended the afternoon session of the Community Study, these thoughts would be equally improbable. Many would find it hard to believe that is happening in Worcester.

The team from Worcester came to the conference as an additional Community Study at the suggestion of participants from the Harvard School of Public Health who knew of the community, its strengths, and its problems. The group agreed to come and work on the difficult task they were facing, which they presented for consideration and discussion.

Goals for a Worcester School Health Program

1. Establish links with private and institutional care providers in the community to ensure that each pupil has a regular source of primary care (medical and dental).
2. Improve services delivered within the school setting, emphasizing:
    a. delivery of minimum services required by regulation;
    b. early identification of health problems through individual assessment;
    c. coordination in the management of specific health problems; and
    d. provision and coordination of services related to pregnancy, venereal disease, drug abuse/alcoholism, child neglect and abuse, nutrition, learning, and emotional problems.
3. Develop a systemwide, organized program for implementation of Chapter 766 of the state's education law, integrating the health department and school department efforts, skills, and resources. Such a program should include as a minimum:
    a. preschool screening and identification;
    b. parent education;
    c. core evaluations; and
    d. expanded services and coverage in specialized schools.

These goals had been hammered out in several preconference meetings. There was not a great deal of optimism on the part of the liaison staff person as to whether the team would hold together long enough to get to Galveston. The team represented the schools, the public health department, and other interests. Contained within the group was a long-standing interdisciplinary and interagency standoff. The state law created a situation that required that they work together, but it did not require that they like it.

Worcester, Massachusetts, located about 35 miles west of Boston, has a population of approximately 175,000; it is old, eastern, urban, and ethnic. For a resident of the southwest, that describes a pretty foreign environment. Worcester is, however, more similar to more of the United States than the three other cities. It is in a region of rolling, wooded hills, numerous lakes and streams (the city is located on Lake Quinsigamond), and valleys with farms and orchards. Much of the land between Worcester and Boston is a mix of suburban communities, urban sprawl, countryside, and industrial development.

Substantial urban renewal and redevelopment has occurred in Worcester in recent years; its economic life is concentrated in manufacturing, commerce, and services (especially education). The city itself has a land area of 37.16 square miles. The Standard Metropolitan Statistical Area (SMSA) that surrounds it includes 21 towns (in New England, towns and cities have coterminous boundaries; there is no unincorporated county land), and 475 square miles with approximately 344,320 people (1970). The predominating ethnic groups are of French Canadian, Irish, Italian, Swedish, and English origin.

Worcester is an educational center with seven four-year colleges, four junior colleges, a technical institute, and the University of Massachusetts Medical School. Worcester has been hard hit by recession; the unemployment rate is about 12 percent, and the city is classified as an area of substantial unemployment.

The proportion of people of Spanish-speaking or Hispanic origin in the population has been growing in recent years. The city also has areas of very high mobility and population turnover. Overall, as noted, the city is slowly declining in population, a trend characteristic of many old central cities.

There are 28,000 students in 62 public schools in Worcester, with an additional 4,400 in 11 parochial schools. Percentages of minority students are still low for an urban school system, with less than 9 percent being black or of Hispanic origin.

Two attempts have been made to create a joint school department/health department task force for school health in the past. The first, over a decade ago, focused on upgrading sanitary and health conditions in the schools themselves; it was disbanded as problems were solved. The second was formed several years ago as aggressive special education laws were first being proposed in the state, but it lasted only briefly and accomplished little.

The new state special education law (Chapter 766) is now in its second year. Its strong requirements for "core evaluations" and individualized placements for all children with special needs (emphasizing preschool identification, multidisciplinary evaluations, mainstreaming, and parent involvement), coming at a time of budget restraints, has led the schools to attempt to develop cooperative arrangements with external medical and health resources, including the school health program and public health.

At the same time, because of this and other changing factors, the health department contracted with the Harvard School of Public Health in 1975 to do a study of the department's operations and to recommend future changes in goals, procedures, and organization. This report was released in May 1976 and proposed major, but gradual changes in the current school health program.

An informal group on school health, convened by the Department of Public Health, had met four times in the spring prior to the conference. It included representatives of the Department of Public Health, Worcester Public Schools, Worcester Diocese, the city's Office of Human Services, local health centers (Office of Economic Opportunity and private group practice), the University of Massachusetts Medical School at Worcester, and the Harvard School of Public Health. Members from this working group comprised the community study team coming to Galveston. The initial impetus for its creation was the announcement of the possible opportunity to participate in the conference and to use that situation to develop a community program for change.

At the conference, the Worcester team offered a well-developed presentation on its community and stated their problem in terms of goals (previously stated). The audience immediately recognized the interdisciplinary conflict as the basis for the problem. After some discussion on specifics of the situation presented and many suggestions on approach, the session adjourned without resolving anything. The members of the audience had made several observations concerning the behavior of team members, which exposed the schism among them. As the session ended, the team promised that they would meet that evening and try to reach an agreeable conclusion for approaching the problem. They assured the audience participants that they were "not enemies."

The next morning the team members individually reported to the sessions on various phases of a most difficult two and one-half hour meeting the night before, which had resulted in an unexpected meeting of the minds. Much to the astonishment of the participants, the team had come together and organized the basic structure for a School Health Council with the team members as the core. They planned to add medical and consumer representation on returning to Worcester. Using the council as the method, they had worked out steps to be taken toward the goals presented. The team was highly pleased with itself and with the results. It credited the setting, the tone of the conference, and the input and observations from the audience for the success they had experienced, along with the fact that they were away from home and had found themselves forced to face one another and make some real plans.

Everyone recognized the pitfalls of leaving the conference on an "emotional high." The real test would occur on returning home. By all reports, this team has been amply tested and has retained its ability to tackle difficult problems and work them through.

An initial obstacle reported was the decision to take two nurses from the health department to work with the schools in evaluating children requiring special education. This accomplished, the council turned to the larger task of developing goals and objectives for a comprehensive school health program.

One and one-half years after the conference, the council is beginning to detail a pilot project encompassing these goals and objectives. This project will be piloted in two schools, utilizing a decentralized approach to school health services. Each school will have a school health team reflecting the needs of that school and its neighborhood. The school principal, the school nurse, a part-time physician, and a school health educator will function as the core group on this team. Additional personnel such as counselors, special education teachers, and parents will be brought in as needed. The council also plans to begin a task analysis on the nurses and physicians currently working in the schools. This analysis will aid in determining the type of personnel needed and additional educational requirements for any job changes.

The Worcester team has remained largely intact since the conference. Although the members have changed positions within the city administration, no one has left the team. A strengthening feature has been the assignment of a staff person from the human services department. Problems continue to arise, but the council has retained its problem-solving capacity, demonstrated as recently as two months ago. A major obstacle still facing the council is the issue of decentralizing control of the health department nurses. They will become more independent, and guidance will be necessary at a more technical level.

The School Health Council finds itself revamping a traditional service. The ability of the council to work within the city administration could, in the long run, aid the program and avoid duplication of services by community agencies.

In reviewing the Worcester experience, it can be seen that, once again, a community team finds its way by working on an organizational structure. In this case, the dynamics of the group process became obvious for all to see. Both the skills of the facilitator, as well as the participation of the larger group, helped the dramatic breakthrough to come. All the resources necessary were *already present* in the community and in the people, and synergy occurred—the whole is greater than the sum of its parts.

COMMUNITY STUDY: HIDALGO, TEXAS

Hidalgo is another world, another culture, perhaps even another century. To go to Hidalgo is to go back in time, at least to the 1930s, when everyone was poor and many communities functioned on a basic level. Despite the poverty, the images that many visitors carry away are the gentle cohesion of the community, its traditional hospitality, and most of all, its resourcefulness and optimism.

Hidalgo was the first community approached by the conference steering committee to consider becoming a Community Study. It is typical of Hidalgo that the project became a community affair. The mayor chaired the Community Study team and was joined by the superintendent of schools, city councilmen, school board members, businessmen, teachers, and parents. The whole conference steering committee traveled to Hidalgo, and no one has forgotten the experience.

Hidalgo, Texas, seven miles south of McAllen in the lower Rio Grande valley, functions as a gateway to Mexico. Situated on the Rio Grande, historic Hidalgo has an updated population estimate of 2,500 people. By contrast, Reynosa, its sister city across the river in Mexico, is a rapidly growing metropolis with 185,000 residents.

When the team arrived, it was easy to see the results of the last four years. Hidalgo has been getting a facelift. All the one-time dirt streets are now paved and have new curbs and street lights. Before the streets were paved, new sewage and storm drainage systems were laid, and modern sewer and water plants built. A new city hall has been erected, as has a fire station. The municipal law enforcement department has been expanded. A sound community building is neatly kept for meetings, receptions, and bimonthly clinics held by the county health department. A new health clinic, which will also house the child development center and branch library, was being built across from city hall to provde a place to house more continuous health care for the people of Hidalgo. Resources to build the clinic were easier to come by than will be those for health manpower and health services.

Down the street from the municipal building, a city park was under construction with underground facilities. The pool facilities, another example of innovative use of available resources, were completed and ready for summer use, as was the community pavilion, complete with kitchen. In the meantime, trees and grass had been planted. A statue of Father Miguel Hidalgo has found a permanent home at the city park. It was recently presented to the city of Hidalgo by the governor of Tamaulipas, the neighboring state in Mexico. The bronze figure represents the pride of Hidalgo and links the past to the ever-moving present. The statue has a view of city hall, the school, and the street that both buildings face. Esperanza Street is appropriately named, for Hidalgo's future rests on *esperanza*— hope. And the hope is invested in the children, the future generation. (After being in Hidalgo, one tends to talk like that.)

All these descriptions are indications of the resourcefulness of the people of Hidalgo and their leadership. Every one of these projects was either underwritten by or received assistance from the many programs available to economically deprived communities. By careful planning and wise use of available local resources, the city has been able to make excellent use of grants and other programs.

One of the many difficulties about being a poor community is that you must work on problems for which resources or funds can be found, not necessarily on the problems that are most important. One of the outstanding problems in this poor community was health care; a second one was upgrading the schools. To look at school health in Hidalgo was to look at every problem of a poor rural population, with education, language, and cultural hurdles to overcome.

To live in Hidalgo means most likely that one is poor and works in agriculture. These figures for the 1975-76 school year tell the story well: grades covered—kindergarten to eighth; number of students—991; percentage of Spanish surnames—95 percent; percentage of resident aliens—27.2 percent; number of students using bus—443; number of teachers—43; and number of children receiving free lunches—929.

In 1976 approximately 1,200 children attended school in Hidalgo and in nearby communities for grades 9 to 12 (these returned with the completion of the new high school in 1977). The elementary and middle grades were offered by the Hidalgo Independent School District, which stretches 25 miles wide into the county. Most of the school district area is outside the Hidalgo city limits and is strictly rural—with fields and houses interspersed. The rural neighborhoods in the school district outside Hidalgo are called *colonias,* which are plagued with the problems of substandard housing, lack of indoor plumbing, inadequate water supply, and dirt streets and roads that flood after almost any rain.

Without any local news media, the families who live in the colonias skirting Hidalgo gain information about school from notices posted at the neighborhood stores or *tiendas.* But what the colonias really signify are a rural life for so many children who are not touched directly by the events in the city.

Much of the community life in Hidalgo is still face-to-face: informal relationships, extended family, and social life centered predominantly around church and home. But lest there be a tendency to romanticism, labor is unskilled, 60 percent of the families are in poverty, and real misery exists.

There is no question that the community leadership saw the National School Health Conference as another opportunity for possible resources for the health needs. Planning for attending the conference became a major event in the life of the community. After the initial visit, a member of the conference steering committee made a number of trips during the months prior to the conference. The preparation as outlined in the guidelines (see the Appendix) literally carried the community team through a planning process for school health. The needs were so basic, however, and the resources so limited, that the group had difficulty settling on a reasonable problem with some chance of a solution.

The team came to the conference after considerable preparation. Developing the slide show was an important activity and showing it in the community was a major event. Finally, the problem on which the team settled was stated in the following questions: *What kind of school health program will be needed to meet the needs of our community (in terms that have meaning for our community); and How would we in Hidalgo Independent School District go about setting up the kind of school health program being discussed at this conference—how to start, first phases, timetable?*

Once in Galveston, the team members' enthusiastic participation in all the events of the conference gave an added dimension to everyone's experience. In turn, they absorbed everything, trying to relate what they were learning to the realities of Hidalgo.

At the Community Study session the team made a good presentation, and during the discussion that followed the participants worked with the team very well; many suggestions came forth. The specter of the lack of resources in the school and community, however, haunted every effort to work out the details of a basic school health plan. Several times the work ground to a halt when one of the team members would get stuck on the question, "How are we going to get the money for that?" The attempt to design the kind of program to meet the needs kept running to the reality of "what can we expect to do with what we have and what we are likely to get in the future?" The participants were really able to visualize what they were up against, and it tended to be overwhelming.

The Hidalgo team left the conference with numerous lists of things to do, but without a focused plan for school health. They took with them the knowledge that they had done a good job and had made a fine contribution to the conference, both individually and as a team. The facilitator of the session was probably the most frustrated, feeling that the team had not been given what they came for.

In the months that followed, not a great deal of information filtered back to the members of the conference steering committee. It was known that the School of Allied Health Sciences of UTMB was following up on plans for a screening effort for the schools. Most important, it was learned that the community study team had been formalized with a

School Health Service Advisory Committee and was working with representatives from UTMB.

A year and a half later, the resourcefulness of the leadership of Hidalgo, stimulated by what they learned in Galveston, has led to an amazing number of improvements in the community and schools concerning the health of the children. When the team came to Galveston, the one health professional in the community, the school nurse, had left with no replacement in sight. There is now a nurse who spends three days in the elementary school and two days in the newly opened high school. She has been joined by three aides and one home health agent doing home visits. Physician coverage for the newly opened community health clinic has been scheduled at regular times during the week.

There is a public health nurse in the community health clinic all day, five days a week, providing well child care, prenatal guidance, health education, immunizations, nutrition education, etc. When the Hidalgo team came to Galveston for the conference, public health was served in the community only twice a month on Tuesdays. Health education programs also are being presented at PTA meetings. Recognition of the need for a full-time elementary school counselor resulted from participation in the Community Study session. This position has been created and filled.

There is no doubt that participation in the conference was an important event and focused the community's attention on health. It opened the way for a multidisciplinary team of students and faculty from UTMB to conduct an extensive screening program in the elementary school. Medical students, physician's assistants, pediatric nurse practitioners, physical therapists, occupational therapists, and medical technology students, with faculty supervision, have screened over 700 children in three comprehensive efforts. Follow-up care for all children with identified problems has been completed. Reports on the health status of the children of Hidalgo has been presented to the school board.

High school students have formed a health club and obtained free toothpaste and brushes to do demonstrations. These students helped with the screening programs, providing valuable assistance. While at the programs, they gave demonstrations on dental hygiene for the children being screened. At the latest screening program, over 60 percent of the parents participated. Finally, developmental screening has been started in the colonias for preschool children.

There is no doubt that much still remains to be done in Hidalgo. Community members involved in the conference expressed concern over the attitudes in Hidalgo with regard to school health services. They felt the provision of services by the school was not yet a high enough priority with many of the community residents. Also cited as barriers to gaining school health services were the lack of professional personnel residing in the community (especially doctors), the lack of funds for an ongoing program, and a general lack of information and communication within the health system. Planning continues to be episodic and incremental. But something vital has happened in Hidalgo, and it will continue to happen.

In Hidalgo the schools and the community worked together, demonstrating a little of what can be accomplished when school health is involved in the community, as well as when the community is involved in school health.

OBSERVATIONS

At this point, after looking at the Community Study sessions, it is still not possible to assess fully the value of the National School Health Conference, nor to identify all that was learned. Some interesting things are beginning to emerge from the follow-up. Maybe the best thing to do is list some of these so they will be available for future reference. Hindsight could make some of these things a little clearer as time goes by.*

- In the Community Study sessions, each community focused on an organizational problem and how to bring about change. This says something about a need to learn and utilize the new technologies of organizational development and systems change. Intersystem arrangements seem to be where school health lives best.
- It might not be important or necessary to develop a "theoretical structure" for school health, or even to try to define it. In fact, these efforts could actually be harmful. Definition means limitation. Perhaps school health is not ready for these kinds of limits.
- It is interesting how important sheer information is, how much people need to know about what is going on and what works, how strongly groups are still wrestling with roles, and how surprised everyone always is at the difficulties experienced in trying to *communicate* across discipline boundaries, let alone *work* together.
- School health people do not seem to know a lot about planning, nor are they comfortable thinking in goal-directed terms. Perhaps it is because they have so little opportunity— a point worth exploring.
- "Family" and "community" remain items of concern and ambiguity. How professionals in school health can enlarge unanswered challenge.

---

*Several of these items, along with points raised in other chapters, receive further development in Chapter 7.

- Conferences, as an activity, seem to hold some promise as a method of intervention. State level conferences in school health could be a method of choice to explore next.

As the teams interacted with the participants, new ideas came forth. The participants, serving as consultants to the team, were able to provide a variety of expertise as well as a perspective of objectivity, which the teams sorely needed. During these sessions, the idea that people are the most important resource began to come into its own. People saw a little of what can happen when an interdisciplinary team attacks a problem. Some identified it as synergy in action.

Each team emerged with a set of possible steps to use in tackling their problem and with many suggestions for solutions to the larger issues they faced. Assessing the results of the Community Study sessions is complicated. To say the least, the interaction in all four of them was spirited, and the teams themselves found them to be most useful. A poignant comment was overheard in the early evening from a woman who had been in school health services for many years. She said, "Watching the teams in action, I realize that I don't remember a time in our schools when people representing all those different areas sat down to work on a problem together."

The participants had come with few expressed expectations in the area of how social systems change. Many came out of the Community Study sessions aware that they had witnessed something extremely important, though few could express exactly what that was. As subsequent events have borne out, they had, in fact, participated in changes in the lives of those communities.

Chapter 6

Budgeting and Financing of School Health Services

COST OF SCHOOL HEALTH SERVICES

School health services are receiving increased attention from school officials, health professionals, and taxpayers. School officials are interested in making the best use of limited school health dollars while providing the required health services. Health professionals see school health services as a potential locus of improved child health care and see new opportunities to coordinate school health care with other health services. Taxpayers and parents of school-children are requesting justification of continued expenditures that contribute to ever-rising school budgets.

Although no significant movement is apparent in the United States to provide a full range of health services under the school roof, an increasing amount of experimentation is occurring to expand health services in the school setting. Yet despite a renewed interest in school health services, data concerning their cost are inadequate.

Substantial sums are spent annually for school health services in the United States. During the 1970-71 school year, expenditures for school health and attendance services were $369 million.[1] These expenditures had risen to $452 million by the 1973-74 school year, an increase of 23 percent in only three years.[2] Although representing only 1 percent of the total current expenditures for public school systems, expenditures for school health kept pace with the rise of total expenditures of local public school systems during the same period. Total expenditures for schools rose from $45.5 billion in 1970-71 to $56.2 billion in 1973-74, an increase of 23 percent.[3] Actually, the estimates for school health are substantially less than total expenditures. School lunch programs, nutrition services, and psychological counseling are not included in these totals. If they were, total expenditures estimates for school health-related services would have exceeded $1 billion in 1976.

A summary of school health expenditures by region and by system size indicates that those expenditures are increasing in each geographical region (Table 6-1). The Plains and Great Lakes region has increased its expenditures at a faster rate than have other regions when adjusted to match enrollment increases. The smallest school systems, those with enrollments under 2,500, have increased their expenditures the least during a recent four-year period.[4]

Expenditures for school health per pupil remain low. The average expenditure by school system per pupil was $8.21 during the 1970-71 school year, and $10.36 during the 1973-74 school year. In comparison, the National Center for Health Statistics estimated the annual cost of health care for a child in the United States to be $165.00 in 1971.

By expenditure category, the largest expenditures in school health are for personnel, mainly nurses. The estimated number of full-time equivalents of school health personnel in public school systems is 25,000; 17,000 of whom are school nurses.[5] The average expenditure per child for school health services in several states is shown in Table 6-2 and is related to the estimated nurse-student ratio.

Although total expenditures for school health in the United States are large, individual school systems must carefully budget limited resources. Yet, at present, few programs are using a disciplined approach to budgets. In the following pages, managers of school-related health services are offered relatively simple approaches to budgeting and financing. First, a basic distinction must be made: budgeting is the process of translating goals and objectives of a program into projected costs; financing is the process of obtaining revenues or grants to meet such costs.

BUDGETING SCHOOL HEALTH SERVICES

The first step in the budgeting process is to list the basic assumptions on which a program is to be developed. These assumptions should be agreed on by all persons responsible for carrying out the program before it is launched. For example, one assumption might be that the program will provide services to all children in the school district regardless of income or alternative source of health care. Or an assumption might be that money currently in school health budgets will be reallocated to

Table 6-1 Current Expenditures of Local Public School Systems Allocable to Pupil Costs, for Attendance and Health Services and by Enrollment Size of System and Region: United States, 1970-74

Enrollment Size of System and Region	Attendance and Health Services (in thousands of dollars)		
	70-71	72-73	73-74
Total— United States	$361,333	$428,724	$451,954
25,000 or more enrollment	129,857	163,165	170,879
North Atlantic	42,423	58,408	*
Great Lakes and Plains	39,178	50,634	*
Southeast	12,338	13,848	*
West and Southwest	35,918	40,276	*
10,000-24,999 enrollment	67,647	71,991	79,176
North Atlantic	31,962	34,336	*
Great Lakes and Plains	12,565	12,593	*
Southeast	5,835	8,273	*
West and Southwest	17,285	16,790	*
5,000-9,999 enrollment	62,545	75,230	76,843
North Atlantic	33,948	42,469	*
Great Lakes and Plains	10,279	11,149	*
Southeast	9,401	10,330	*
West Southwest	8,916	11,282	*
2,500-4,999 enrollment	50,990	60,184	63,880
North Atlantic	29,144	36,647	*
Great Lakes and Plains	7,705	8,558	*
Southeast	6,896	6,849	*
West and Southwest	7,246	8,131	*
Under 2,500 enrollment	50,293	58,153	61,176
North Atlantic	27,532	28,161	*
Great Lakes and Plains	10,479	14,299	*
Southeast	4,031	6,096	*
West and Southwest	8,251	9,597	*

*Information not available

Sources: *Statistics of Local Public School Systems Finance 1970-71* (NCES 75-149);
Statistics of Local Public School Systems Finance 1972-73 (NCES 76-156);
Statistics of Local Public School Systems Finance 1973-74 (NCES 76-157).

Table 6-2 U.S. School Health Expenditures and Staff 1973-74*

	Total Enrollment**	Total Expenditures for Attendance and Health Services** (thousands of dollars)	Expenditure Per Pupil in ADA**	Nurse/ Nurses** Pupils**
Alabama	770,739	2,481	3.43	— 1:
Alaska	82,505	540	10.28	42 1:1,964
Arizona	521,240	6,438	14.34	433 1:1,203
Arkansas	450,114	1,597	4.07	81 1:5,556
California	4,459,328	35,869	8.08	1,989 1:2,241
Colorado	573,154	6,039	10.79	217 1:2,641
Connecticut	667,088	7,841	12.23	†
Delaware	132,940	1,966	14.72	171 1:777
D.C.	136,036	6,489	47.55	†
Florida	1,537,952	2,987	1.95	56 1:2,746
Georgia	1,085,881	4,435	4.72	†
Hawaii	178,511	6,381	36.15	†
Idaho	189,133	707	3.99	45 1:4,202
Illinois	2,320,672	35,175	17.05	1,233 1:1,882
Indiana	1,207,420	7,814	6.82	533 1:2,265
Iowa	631,132	4,148	6.95	352 1:1,792
Kansas	460,896	2,630	5.68	270 1:1,707
Kentucky	709,764	4,645	6.94	85 1:8,350
Louisiana	842,152	3,825	4.52	283 1:2,975
Maine	245,467	1,076	4.64	74 1:3,317
Maryland	911,097	11,137	13.59	—
Massachusetts	1,205,142	18,082	15.44	1,234 1:976
Michigan	2,123,611	14,875	6.72	—
Minnesota	900,377	9,187	11.01	483 1:1,864
Mississippi	519,786	1,811	3.46	101 1:5,146
Missouri	1,019,803	7,036	7.64	611 1:1,669
Montana	172,045	1,883	9.94	—
Nebraska	323,211	2,972	9.83	107 1:3,020
Nevada	135,406	862	6.43	51 1:2,655
New Hampshire	171,482	1,845	11.22	188 1:912
New Jersey	1,481,605	32,352	21.94	—

*1973-74 is the latest year for which all information is available

**Total enrollment—enrollment in public elementary and secondary schools by state, Fall 1973. Total expenditures for attendance and health services—current expenditures by local public school systems allocable to pupil costs 1973-74. Expenditure per pupil in ADA—current expenditures per pupil in average daily membership in local public school systems 1973-74. Nurses—nurses employed by local education agencies by state (in full-time equivalents). Nurse/pupils—ratio of full-time nursing equivalents to total student enrollment by state.

†States did not report these data.

Table 6-2 Continued

	Total Enrollment**	Total Expenditures for Attendance and Health Services** (thousands of dollars)	Expenditure Per Pupil in ADA**	Nurses**	Nurse/ Pupils**
New Mexico	283,550	1,784	6.67	144	1:1,969
New York	3,449,430	71,480	20.72	2,299	1:1,500
North Carolina	1,173,415	4,012	3.57	—	
North Dakota	138,302	351	2.64	2	1:69,151
Ohio	2,378,349	18,231	7.96	702	1:3,387
Oklahoma	600,948	2,630	4.51	135	1:4,451
Oregon	476,518	1,575	3.37	83	1:5,741
Pennsylvania	2,321,437	49,177	22.41	2,280	1:1,035
Rhode Island	184,624	1,526	8.55	—	
South Carolina	626,914	3,510	5.64	130	1:4,822
South Dakota	157,522	466	2.97	—	
Tennessee	902,704	3,873	4.62	95	1:9,502
Texas	2,782,151	25,258	9.56	1,250	1:2,225
Utah	305,800	1,196	4.11	45	1:6,795
Vermont	106,236	941	9.57	101	1:1,051
Virginia	1,085,295	6,854	6.49	350	1:3,100
Washington	788,324	6,131	8.26	248	1:3,178
West Virginia	409,184	2,864	7.03	103	1:3,972
Wisconsin	987,022	4,056	4.59	112	1:8,812
Wyoming	85,391	916	10.94 (est.)	62	1:1,377

**Total enrollment—enrollment in public elementary and secondary schools by state, Fall 1973. Total expenditures for attendance and health services—current expenditures by local public school systems allocable to pupil costs 1973-74. Expenditure per pupil in ADA—current expenditures per pupil in average daily membership in local public school systems 1973-74. Nurses—nurses employed by local education agencies by state (in full-time equivalents). Nurse/pupils—ratio of full-time nursing equivalents to total student enrollment by state.

reorganization of services. A negotiated agreement on a list of basic assumptions in advance of a program's development ensures that vested interests will not try to continue traditional elements of school health if an agreement has been made to reorganize the services. Too often, programs try to maintain the established services while grafting on additional services, a practice that is more costly than total reorganization of the services from the beginning.

The next step in the budgeting process is to design the program in a manner that will facilitate identification of the individual elements of cost. Four steps are involved in this process: (1) define the goals and objectives of a program; (2) profile the characteristics of the population to be served; (3) distinguish among cost elements related to service, management, training, or research; and (4) develop a realistic work plan so cost elements can be phased into the budget at the rate at which they occur.

Defining Goals and Objectives

Long-term goals and short-term objectives should be described to determine line-item costs. Budgets should be based on the individual line-items and not be constructed from available funding.

For example, if a long-range program goal is to promote health and to prevent health problems in schoolchildren, an intermediate objective would be to ensure that all schoolchildren are immunized against common diseases. Cost elements such as salaries required to pay personnel dispensing the immunizations, laboratory fees, and supplies would then be anticipated.

A second long-term goal might be the expansion of the role of the school nurse to provide initial assessment and diagnosis of illness. Intermediate objectives would require training programs for the nurses and in-service education for principals and teachers to prepare them for the nurse's expanded role. Specific cost elements, such as the cost of the training program, could then be anticipated only by understanding intermediate objectives. Obtaining individual line items from an analysis of the goals and objectives of a program is tedious, but it is a necessary step for accurate budgeting.

Population Characteristics

Once the goals and objectives of a program are defined, the second step is the development of a profile of the population to be served. For example, immunization rates in a community should be determined. If 95 percent of a school-age population has been immunized before entering school, immunization would not need to be emphasized in the program. The population profile involves subtle elements. For example, knowing how many low income children in a school system are eligible for Medicaid is important. Lack of such information often results in gross miscalculation of available reimbursements for a program.

The size of the population to be served is significant. There are economies of scale in delivering both health and educational services. Just as physicians cannot set up practices with less than a certain population size, it is not feasible to develop a comprehensive system of direct health care for a total population of fewer than 1,000 children. With fewer than 1,000 children, referral and coordination of care would be wiser than direct provision of care. Assuming a sufficient population, appropriate health professional-student ratios can be determined and subsequently translated into cost elements. The most typical nurse-student ratio is 1:1,500. Small school systems of under 5,000 students are least likely to be able to maintain a 1:1,500 nurse-student ratio. J.B. Igoe has suggested that nurse practitioners, as distinguished from traditional school nurses, could be responsible for approximately 1,400 students with the assistance of an aide. This is feasible because in most settings only 25 percent of these students require the nurse practitioner to provide the bulk of care.[6]

In experimental programs around the country, however, ratios vary. The Cambridge, Massachusetts, Pediatric Nurse Practitioner Neighborhood Health Centers have a ratio of 1:700 nurses to children (1974).[7] The Galveston, Texas, school system ratio is similar.[8] An experimental program sponsored by the University of Connecticut Medical Center and the Hartford Board of Education has 1:450 nurses to children (1976).

Conclusive information concerning the most appropriate school physician to student ratio is not available. It is instructive, however, to remember that in general pediatric practice, the average pediatrician averages 139 patient visits weekly in the office. The appropriate physician to student ratio will depend on whether the physician provides the bulk of direct care or is a back-up and referral source for the nurse practitioner. Assuming the presence of nurse practitioners, a full-time physician equivalent per 4,000 children seems to be realistic.

The current health status of the children in a population has implications for budgeting. Too often, the program developer underestimates or overestimates the backlog of medical or dental care which will be required to bring a population of children to a point where preventive health maintenance can be begun. A study of the experience of the federally funded Child and Youth Projects[9] or the Health Start Program[10] can provide information concerning how to determine current health status of children.

Local health departments, community pediatricians, and dentists will have general indications as to the health status of the community. Once such health profiles are established, some estimates can be made as to the anticipated volume of care. It should be considered, however, that with the presence of a nurse practitioner in the school, the volume of care demanded might actually increase as previously undetected health problems are identified and care is initiated.[11, 12]

In general, the data available concerning the morbidity of school-age children are limited. The prevalence of common childhood medical problems among Head Start children, however, has been compiled (Table 6-3).

The socioeconomic characteristics of a population are useful to determine the possible sources of reimbursement. Each program should develop a strategy to ensure that children who are potentially eligible for third-party reimbursement are registered for such reimbursement.

Distinguish Among Service, Management, Training, and Research Costs

Because any service program has many goals, budgets must be developed in such a way as to distinguish costs that are related to service from costs that are related to management, training, or research. This becomes critically important when the program is evaluated. In budget-

---

Table 6-3 Incidence of Pediatric Health Problems Detected in Head Start Children

Complete eye evaluation because of failed screening test	10.0%
Eyeglasses	1.0%
Eye surgery	<0.1%
Complete hearing evaluation	1-2.0%
Follow-up of positive tuberculin test	1-4.0%
Iron deficiency anemia	10-40.0%
Heart murmur requiring special evaluation	1-4.0%
Urinary infection	0.5%
Inguinal hernia	0.25-1.0%
Skin disease	2-5.0%
Asthma, hay fever	2-5.0%
Seizures	1-2.0%
Impaired learning requiring diagnostic evaluation (may be included in psychological services)	2-10.0%
Behavioral abnormality requiring diagnostic evaluation (may be included in psychological services, may be same children as those with learning problems)	2-5.0%
Tonsils, circumcisions, umbilical hernias	0-1.0%

Note: The cost of care to remedy defects discovered in the health evaluations can be estimated by multiplying the average cost in a community of providing certain common types of medical services by the estimated number of children who will require such services. The average cost can be estimated by the health director in each community. The percentage of children who will require each service can be estimated from the previous experience in each community. The table lists the most common defects requiring treatment and estimates of their frequency based on Head Start experience and on other studies.

Source: *Project Head Start. Health Services* (Washington, D.C., U.S. Government Printing Office, 1971), p. 23.

ing for residency training for physicians, for example, only by distinguishing between the time that the faculty devotes to training and that devoted to service can accurate estimates be made of what the program costs. School-related health service programs could appear inordinately expensive to school boards if the costs related to research or education components are not carefully distinguished from costs related to delivery of care.

Development of Realistic Work Plans

Work plans should anticipate the length of time required to negotiate for reimbursement from third-party sources, to obtain funding from private philanthropies, and to negotiate with the board of education, unions, or community health groups. Perhaps the most frequent error in program development is premature staffing; the result is a heavy front-end cost to a project. A realistic lead time for almost every project that plans to deliver health services is at least 18 months. Obviously, much activity can occur during the interim. In school health, for example, the training of the nurses should occur during this 18-month period.

In summary, once the goals and objectives are clearly stated, salary costs, costs of materials, space requirements, and so on can be estimated. Profiling the population will provide the dimensions of expected utilization of services. Distinguishing among elements related to service, management, training, or research aspects of the program will provide a basis for the most accurate evaluation of a program. Finally, realistic work plans allow a clear appraisal of how various costs should be phased into a budget over the life of a program.

FINANCING SCHOOL-RELATED HEALTH SERVICES

Financing is the process of securing income to pay for the expenditures required by a program. In the school health program, the most usual sources of income will be direct or indirect contributions to school health from tax revenues through budgets of local health departments or boards of education. Other sources of income are grants or contracts from private or public agencies and direct reimbursement from third-party insurers.

Sources of income should be identified at least 18 months in advance of the operational date of a program. The phasing of different aspects of the program, such as expanding the scope of services to include dental care or the development of a health education curriculum, will depend on the timing of the receipt of revenues.

There are several "facts of life" in financing: the need for multiple sources of funds, the need for protection from negative cash flow, the need to assess realistically potential fiscal self-sufficiency, the need to develop a reimbursement mechanism, and the need to minimize capital expenditures.

Multiple sources of funds are needed because no single agency can be expected to pay for all costs associated with a comprehensive school health program. Throughout the social service sector, private and public funds must be used together to "package" programs. Not only are the resources of public and private agencies limited with respect to what they can contribute, but also public and private sector investors welcome partners in any new venture. This minimizes the risk to any one party. Consequently, the school health innovators should try to get as broad a base of support as possible and as early as possible. Broad-based support also protects the program itself by ensuring its financial independence from any one source of financing. Unexpected fluctuations in income can be minimized by seeking multiple sources of funding.

Cash flow is the rate at which cash is available to pay bills. The health sector is particularly vulnerable to negative cash flow. (This means that cash is required to pay salaries, for example, faster than the rate at which cash is made available to the program.) Any health program should anticipate such problems.

Few school-related health services programs will ever be fiscally self-sufficient. Therefore, in planning the financing of such programs, those elements that will require continued grant support should be distinguished from those elements for which reimbursement can be obtained over time. Program developers should seriously consider using the services of existing agencies rather than starting services for which reimbursement can never be obtained.

Finally, innovative school health programs should attempt to minimize capital expenditures. Securing income for capital formation is the major problem of private industry in the United States and is not limited to the "grant economy." It will be very difficult for school health programs during the next decade to obtain funds for the capital expenditures that will be needed to construct health-related facilities. Therefore, school health programs should minimize the need for new capital expenditures and maximize the use of existing space and leased or borrowed equipment. Studies have shown that investing in capital equipment for school health programs is unlikely to be a wise investment, unless such services are made available after school hours to the larger community.[13]

In addition to the previously discussed "facts of life" of financing innovations of school health services, sources of financing for health will be found to differ from traditional sources of financing for all local public school system expenditures. In general, public school budgets are financed mainly through local and intermediate sources (for example, counties) and least by federal sources (Table 6-4). For example, of the $529 billion received by local public school systems in the 1973-74 school year, 54 percent was derived from local and intermediate sources, 39 percent from state sources, and only 7 percent from federal sources. Traditionally, school health services appear to have been financed in roughly the same way. This is consistent with the traditional separation of federal involvement in the financing of local school health.

The financing of health services in general, however, has gone the other way in the United States. Since 1965 when Medicaid and Medicare were introduced, the bulk of public assistance for health care to the population is derived from federal support. Of the total Medicaid bill (a federal-state cost sharing program) which was $3.7 billion in 1968 and $6.5 billion in 1971, the federal share was 49 percent and 58 percent, respectively.[14] The inescapable conclusion is that although total revenue receipts for schools will continue to come from local and state sources, revenues for financing expanded or improved school *health* services out of public dollars will come from federal reimbursement. This requires a different frame of mind for the administrator used to working with local budget committees. He or she will now have to learn how to tap federal reimbursement mechanisms.

Although the possibility of calling upon previously untapped federal dollars to pay for school health has been raised, reallocation of current school dollars must also be considered in the financing of any school health program. This can be very difficult because reallocation means that existing programs must truly become part of the innovation, which might require elimination or significant change in the positions of per-

---

Table 6-4 Revenue Receipts of Local Public School Systems by Source of Funds

(thousands of dollars)

	1970-71	Percentage	1973-74	Percentage
Total	$42,423,838	100	$52,914,027	100
Local and intermediate	23,355,369	55	28,313,374	54
State	15,783,663	37	20,639,752	39
Federal	3,284,806	8	3,811,623	7

sons long established in their roles. Innovation can be painful in one's own backyard, but true costs cannot be measured if duplication is permitted to continue.

Sources of Funds for School-Related Health Services Programs

Private and public funding programs for school-related health services programs are fragmented. Private funding can be obtained from foundations on a one-by-one basis. Program directors should look locally for private foundation support while keeping in mind that private philanthropy's interest lies in providing developmental support rather than funding operational deficits. Foundations are also becoming more concerned that the developmental support they provide does not result in launching programs for which there is no subsequent local support. Program developers should be prepared to present convincing arguments that a school-related health services program will improve the coordination of care and is not repetitious of services already being provided.

In general, however, private funding is not likely to be a major source of funding school health. Nationally, private philanthropy accounts for less than 4.2 percent of all expenditures for health, and this percentage is decreasing every year.

Federal Funding of School Health Programs

Groups developing a school-related health services program should consider federal funding for some elements of the program. To date, there has been little in the way of direct federal support for school health programs. This should not be surprising considering the traditional separation of the federal government from involvement in local school services. There are, however, several categorical grant programs which could provide some monies for elements of school-related programs. The following is a brief description of the major programs that should be explored for sources of funding. Expanded information on each of these programs is available in the *Federal Catalogue of Domestic Assistance.*[15]

*Department of Agriculture—Special Supplemental
Food Program for Women, Infants
and Children (WIC Program)*

The objective of this program is to supply nutritious foods to pregnant or lactating women, infants, and children through local, public, or nonprofit private health agencies. Most state health departments participate

Table 6-5 Demonstration Projects in School Health and Nutrition Services for Children from Low Income Families Effective January 1976

Location of Project

Nutrition Division
Center for Developmental and Learning
  Disorders
University of Alabama
Birmingham, Alabama 35233
(205) 934-5401

Tucson School District #1
1010 East Tenth Street
Tucson, Arizona 85719
(602) 791-6243

Orleans Parish School Board
Thomy LaFon Elementary School
2601 Seventh Street
New Orleans, Louisiana 70115
(504) 899-2338

Harrison School
1500 Fourth Avenue North
Room 101
Minneapolis, Minnesota 55405
(612) 377-9802

District Health Resource Center
1070 East 104 Street
Brooklyn, New York
(212) 241-5761

Terry Mill School
797 Fayetteville Road, S.E.
Atlanta, Georgia 30316
(404) 373-7747

Crispus Attucks School
1865 71st Street
Cleveland, Ohio 44115
(216) 881-3777

School Health & Nutrition Services
Division of Health Administration
Providence School Department
Camden One School
60 Camden Avenue
Providence, Rhode Island 02908
(401) 351-3424

Source: Department of Health, Education, and Welfare, Office of Education.

---

in this program, and it should be possible for school-related health service programs serving pregnant teen-agers to obtain food supplements for them under this program.

Office of Education of HEW—School Health and
Nutrition Services for Children from Low Income
Families (School Leadership in Coordinating Health Services)

New funding for this program is no longer available. A listing of the demonstration projects funded by the Office of Education is given in Table 6-5.

The program was designed for children who attended Title I Elementary and Secondary Education Act (ESEA) School in kindergarten or grades one through six who came from families with income not exceeding one of the following: Office of Economic Opportunity Poverty Line Index, the State Title XIX Medicaid Standards, or the Department of Welfare Statewide Standards for Financial Assistance.

The programs, which vary considerably across the country, were designed to demonstrate ways to organize systems of comprehensive health and education services by improving the coordination of existing health and educational resources in a community. School systems took the lead in developing the mechanisms of coordination. Although funding is not available, valuable information may be obtained from the Division of Drug and Nutrition and Health Programs Office of Education with respect to the experience of these programs.

Office of Education of HEW—Educationally Deprived Children— Migrants (Title I Migrants)

This program is designed to expand and improve educational programs to meet the special needs of children of migratory agricultural workers or migratory fishermen. The program funds can be used to identify and meet specific needs of migrant children through remedial instruction, health, nutrition, psychological services, cultural development, and prevocational training counseling. Eligibility is through each state, and children are required to have documentation that they indeed have parents or guardians who were migrants as recently as five years earlier. There is a matching requirement for this program. Several school health programs have made use of these funds for particular segments of their population; others are encouraged to consider this as an option.

Office of the Secretary of HEW—Child Development— Child Abuse and Neglect Prevention and Treatment (Child Abuse)

The objective of this program is to provide support to state, local, and voluntary agencies or organizations that are trying to strengthen their ability to develop programs that will prevent, identify, and treat child abuse and neglect. Indirectly, such monies might serve to strengthen school health programs that are interested in addressing the problems of child abuse.

Health Resources Administration, Public Health Service, HEW—Division of Nursing—Nurse Training Act of 1975

Funding is currently available for traineeships for nurses to become school nurse practitioners at institutions that have received funding from the Division of Nursing. Major limitations on such traineeships are that they normally require full-time attendance during the trainee period. Such funding should not be ignored, however, if there is a possibility that the nurses in a school-related health services program can take advantage of such traineeships.

Center for Disease Control, Public Health Service,
HEW—Childhood Lead-Based Paint Poisoning Control

Funding is available to stimulate communities to develop comprehensive programs of control of lead-based paint poisoning. Public agencies of general local government and agencies of state government which provide direct services are eligible to apply for grants. Several school health programs around the country who suspect that they have young children with lead paint problems have taken advantage of this funding.

Health Services Administration, Public Health Service, HEW—
Maternal and Child Health Research
(Child Health Research Grants Program)

Funding is provided to research projects relating to maternal and child health services or crippled children's services that show promise of substantial contribution to their advancement. Examples of areas that are being investigated include methods of increasing effectiveness of child health programs, especially services for school-age children and for retarded children. State and local governments are included among eligible applicants.

Social and Rehabilitation Service, HEW—
Medical Assistance Program—Medicaid Title XIX)

Most school-related health service programs will find that a certain percentage of children in the school are eligible or potentially eligible for Medicaid reimbursement for medical services received. Medicaid is the federally aided state-option medical assistance program. State Medicaid programs must pay for medical services for everyone who qualifies for federally aided financial assistance under programs for the aged, blind, disabled, or children eligible for AFDC (Aid for Dependent Children). The state can include additional services and can include people who need medical but not financial assistance if they qualify as aged, blind, disabled, or members of families with dependent children. Because state regulations concerning Medicaid vary from state to state, as do the services covered, each school-related health services program would have to study its own potential population and determine how best to secure reimbursement for those children who are referred into a system of medical care and who are eligible for Medicaid services.

In 1967 Congress amended Title XIX to direct attention to the importance of preventive health services for eligible Medicaid children. In 1972 regulations and guidelines were established for the early and periodic screening, diagnosis and treatment (EPSDT) program of Title XIX for children up to 21 years of age. The vigor with which EPSDT programs have been introduced varies considerably from state to state. Potentially, the imaginative developers of school-related health services programs could devise a means by which EPSDT services could be provided to school children in return for reimbursement. The Head Start program already funded several demonstration projects known as Health Start for preschool-aged children to provide them with EPSDT-required services. The potential of tapping EPSDT monies is perhaps the most important avenue of federally funded reimbursement that a school-related health services program should consider.

Manpower Administration, Department of Labor— Comprehensive Employment and Training Programs

The CETA program was designed to provide job training and employment opportunities for economically disadvantaged unemployed and underemployed persons and to assure that training and other services lead to maximum employment opportunities. States, units of general local government having a population of 100,000 or more, and consortia of local government units, at least one of which has a total population of 100,000 or more, are considered eligible for this program. School health programs might consider whether funding may be obtained under CETA to pay salaries of clerical staff or outreach workers who might be involved in an expanded school-related health services program.

STATE FUNDING FOR SCHOOL HEALTH SERVICES

School health is controlled, administered and funded differently in each state. Some states, such as Pennsylvania, have well-developed statewide plans which guide local school districts in the implementation of school health programs. The State school health budget in Pennsylvania is approximately $27 million. An additional amount of approximately the same magnitude is contributed by local school districts to the local programs each year. With these funds, the State of Pennsylvania is beginning to retain school nurses as nurse practitioners, and to reorganize the State's school health system.

The State of California has also begun to implement a program of training school nurses as pediatric nurse practitioners. Numerous local school districts are becoming the locus of screening for EPSDT services.

In the south where public health departments have traditionally been strong, the State of Alabama has secured Appalachian Regional Commission Funds to train public health nurses in the expanded role of nurse practitioners in order to improve school health services.

The State of Massachusetts has begun to investigate the possibility of combining State level budgets for school health with State Medicaid funding in order to carry out the requirements of the 1975 Education for the Handicapped Act, which requires the State to provide school health services, as well as provide the required EPSDT services for eligible children.

The diversity of funding mechanisms at the state level is great. The diversity of funding school health through local sources is even greater. Although the bulk of local funding is derived directly from annual budgetary appropriations, either through the local health department or local board of education budgets, local school health authorities have been able to finance programs through a variety of mechanisms.

In New Orleans, the City Health Department, through its Maternal and Child Health Program, has coordinated with the public school systems to provide EPSDT services to Medicaid eligible children. For services rendered, the schools are reimbursed by the State Welfare Offices via the New Orleans Health Department and the Maternal and Child Health Programs.

In Cambridge, Massachusetts, a different model has emerged. School-*based* ambulatory health services for preschool and school-age children are available. Previously existing well-child stations and the school health services in the eastern section of Cambridge were reorganized so that all services could be provided together. The financing of the program is derived by reallocation of school health budgets, and well-child conference budgets. The program's administrators argue that by reallocating existing resources and replacing retiring school physicians and nurses, the present comprehensive program can be conducted at less cost per child than the previously fragmented system of care. Information released by the program in 1974 stated that the 6,000 children enrolled at that time had 28,228 primary care visits per year at annual per capita costs of $35.15 and total annual costs for primary, secondary, and tertiary care for each child was estimated to be $96.00.

In 1970, Galveston, Texas began a reorganization of its school health services in both its parochial and public schools. A collaboration was begun between the University of Texas Medical Branch and the

Galveston Independent School District. A pediatric faculty member of the Medical School was appointed as medical director of school health services. At the same time a coordinator of the school district health services was also appointed who had a background in school and public health nursing. A demonstration program started soon after for approximately 12,000 students. Funding was obtained from a combination of federal, state, local, and private philanthropic sources. The program successfully convinced the local school board to reallocate existing monies to the demonstration program. This most ambitious program had a working relationship with a children and youth program so that the school health nurse had the capability of referring a child directly into a primary care group practice. Thus, the school system has successfully used existing financial resources to develop an improved health care program.

There are a growing number of similar examples of local school systems taking the initiative to improve school health around the country. What is apparent is that each local system will have to devise its own means of financing and that consistent with the discussion presented earlier in this chapter, the strategy of financing is such that multiple sources of funding are necessary.

REFERENCES

1. G. Kahn, *Statistics of Local Public School System, Finance 1970-71, 1972-73* (National Center for Education Statistics: HEW/Education Division, Washington, D.C., U.S. Government Printing Office).

2. G. Kahn, *Statistics of Local Public School System, Finance 1973-74* (National Center for Education Statistics: HEW/Education Division, Washington, D.C., U.S. Government Printing Office, July 1975).

3. *Ibid.*

4. W. A. Hughes, *Statistics of Local School Systems: Pupils and Staff, Fall 1971* (National Center for Education Statistics: HEW/Education Division).

5. V. Eisner and L.B. Callan, *Dimensions of School Health* (Springfield, Ill.: Charles C. Thomas, 1974).

6. J.B. Igoe, "Should You Become a School Nurse Practitioner?" *Nursing 75* 5, no. 9 (Sept. 1975): 95.

7. P. R. Nader, Cost Analysis Task Force of Galveston Comprehensive School Health Program; personal communication, Jan. 1976.

8. P. Porter, Cost Analysis—Cambridge Pediatric Neighborhood Health Center Annual Report 1974; personal communication, 1975.

9. V. E. Weckwerth, *Final Progress Report: Children and Youth Program and the Systems Development Project* [Minneapolis, Minn.: Minnesota Systems Development Project Inc., 2412 University Avenue S.E., no. 5-7(49), circa 1974].

10. L. M. Vogt, T. White, G. Buchanan, J. Wholey, and R. Zamoff, *Health Start: Final Report of the Evaluation of the Second Year Program* (Washington, D.C., The Urban Institute 964-6, 1973).

11. R. L. Lindahl and W. O. Young, *A Guide to Dental Care for the Early Periodic Screening, Diagnosis, and Treatment Program (EPSDT) Under Medicaid,* prepared by the American Society of Dentistry for Children and the American Academy of Pedodontics for the Social and Rehabilitation Services (Washington, D.C., U.S. Government Printing Office, Aug. 1975).

12. W. K. Frankenburg and A. F. North, *A Guide to Screening for the Early Periodic Screening, Diagnosis and Treatment Program (EPSDT) Under Medicaid,* prepared by the American Academy of Pediatrics for Social and Rehabilitation Service (Washington, D.C., U.S. Government Printing Office, August, 1975).

13. S. Baillie, L. DeWitt, and L. S. O'Leary, *The Potential Role of the School as a Site for Integrating Social Services,* (Syracuse, N.Y.: Education Policy Research Center, Syracuse University Research Corporation, 1972).

14. Louise Russell *et al., Federal Health Spending 1969-74* (Center for Health Policy Studies, National Planning Association, August 1974).

15. Executive Office of the President, Office of Management and Budget, *1977 Catalog of Federal Domestic Assistance* (Washington, D.C., U.S. Government Printing Office, June 1977).

16. G.J. Scott and P.M. Dunn, *Statistics of State School Systems 1973-75* (National Center for Education Statistics: HEW/Education Division, NCES): 76-152.

Chapter 7

Images of the Future

James Williams, M.S.W.

SCHOOL HEALTH—THE CHALLENGE TODAY

The long-established right to education in a democratic society is now inextricably linked to the emerging "right to health" ideal for every citizen. Children with unresolved health problems and without adequate knowledge or ability in their families to maintain wellness cannot develop their full potential in the educational system. Impaired health, therefore, blocks them from full participation in our society. The social, emotional, and financial loss that this represents is being increasingly recognized as a problem that communities must tackle.

HOW DO WE LOOK AT THE FUTURE?

When the National School Health Conference convened in Galveston in June 1976 there were in the audience more than 200 people from all over the United States. This invited group represented a cross section of educational and health professionals actively involved in the present and future of school health. In the hands of this group—and their colleagues at home with whom they will continue to work—could lie the hope of school health in the nation.

If we are going to say that to some degree the future is in our hands, then it becomes important to find out who we are, what we think and what we believe, how we act, and how we look at ourselves and the future. For this reason, the first event of the conference on the first morning was a simple exercise.

An Exercise

That initial exercise was "Imaging the Future." As everyone gathered in the auditorium, they were handed sheets of paper in triplicate and asked to arrange themselves in groups of three. The instructions were that we were all to project ourselves ten years in the future at a gathering in Galveston to review the progress of school health in this decade. We find that everything we had always wanted to happen in school health had come to pass in these ten years. All of our fondest dreams had been realized. We were here in Galveston celebrating the complete success of school health.

Everyone was asked to write down a description of this success.

The reaction to the assignment was as interesting as the results. First, a number of the groups sat in stunned silence trying to comprehend the magnitude of that task they had been assigned. Interaction began to develop as group members tried to write down their images of a future in which all of their hopes and dreams for school health had been realized. During the course of the exercise, amid considerable laughing and joking, many admitted the difficulty of thinking in these terms. Coming as they had from a wide variety of health and educational settings, and working as they did in many different kinds of programs, the group began to realize that it had no unified conception of school health. In other words, *we did not know what success looked like.*

The exercise came to a close when it became clear that everyone had put down all the ideas of which they could think. The orginals of the exercise were handed in, with everyone keeping copies to assist in focusing on the objectives of the conference.[1] Many commented during the course of the conference that the exercise had been an interesting, but sobering, experience.

Results of the Exercise

Analysis of the results of the exercise told us much about ourselves and, perhaps, about the state of school health in general. Certainly, many excellent ideas were embedded in the lists and descriptions that were handed in—ideas that came forth much more clearly as the conference progressed and that formed the basis for some concrete images of the future discussed later on in this chapter. Some problems that the group experienced with the exercise, however, offer considerable insight into the problems we face.

Almost universally, we had difficulty projecting into the future—in other words, we were not at home with one basic skill in planning: setting goals.[2] Responses ranged from an occasional grandiose, utopian comment, such as "Schools have become health service supermarkets for all ages, available to the community on a 24-hour basis," to the completely defeated stance of handing in blank sheets (fortunately rare). The largest number, however, were two- or three-line comments, usually referring to increasing medical services and health teaching. Several of these contained an afterthought about parental involvement.

Several responses simply discribed a law requiring school health (content unspecified). A small minority did not believe that schools should be in any business but education, feeling that health programs had already gone too far and had usurped parental responsibility for the health of children. Several of them would also limit health education in the schools to exclude sex education.

Another large group went into a detailed list of the specific personnel that would constitute a successful school health program. Almost all began by identifying pediatric nurse practitioners (PNPs) in some concentration for all schools, with physician consultation available in some form. Often other personnel were added to the shopping list, such as counselors, psychologists, social workers, and so on. On scarcely any of these lists were there indications of the *purposes* of this group of personnel. It was almost as if they very act of dropping a PNP and a physician into a school would create the successful school health program.

Those respondents who began their lists with programs had almost the same difficulty in identifying specific activities (such as screening for specific diseases) with the goals or scope of the program or how the specific activity fit into a larger whole. In addition, health education was often to be handled by inserting a health educator into the system or by training teachers to be health educators.

Some interesting subtleties emerged in a number of the more detailed responses. Some advocated almost entirely "passive" programs in which students of all ages were seen essentially as patients to be acted upon; that is, to be screened, inoculated, and modified in their behavior. (It is tempting to jump to the conclusion that these responses came essentially from health professionals, but it seems that professionals in education were also capable of desiring passive recipients of services.) Another somewhat smaller group of responses envisioned students as "active" clients, participants who engaged in the process and made decisions as part of the program. "Doing to," "doing for," and "doing with," showed up frequently in the responses, but the last was distinctly in the minority.

Although it was not always possible to distinguish between educators and health care professionals by their responses, each group tended to be locked into its own perspective, listing goals or programs almost exclusively in its own arena. Superordinate goals that transcended the specific areas of interest were rare.

Several other ideas emerged in one form or another. Student participation was occasionally recommended, but without suggestions on how to reconcile it with traditional concepts of professional expertise. "Team" and "interdisciplinary activities" became catchwords, but without an appreciation of how much deliberate effort they require, as was discovered subsequently in many of the conference sessions. (It became all too clear that in some cases, "interdisciplinary" referred to various health disciplines, not to the more complex cross-disciplinary teaming.) Also, a deep ambiguity toward the role of parents showed up often, with parental involvement almost always listed last, and with returning responsibility to parents often sounding almost punitive. Most seemed to agree that parents are needed, but how to get "them" to do what they "should" remained unspecified, for the most part.

Wellness and attitudes toward self, as well as personal responsibility for health, were mentioned often in the responses, although many times these concepts showed up on a list that also included a traditional, passive, disease-oriented view of health programs. The responses to the exercise were not always internally consistent.

One other point of interest is the way the large community figured in the responses: it was rarely mentioned; and whenever it was, outreach staff or advisory bodies, or other possible mechanisms for involving the community, were almost totally absent. About the only way that other aspects of the community figured in the images of the future was in suggestions for better coordination of "other community health and social services." The importance of the community as the social system in which all of our activity occurs was rarely perceived by conference participants at this opening exercise.

Perhaps the most significant characteristic of this group of responses was the almost total lack of any reference to organizational structures to implement the ideas for school health. Out of more than 200 responses, less than ten mentioned a function such as coordination or administration, only four referred to the kind of organizational arrangements necessary to enable the educational and health care systems to interact and to do school health in some form, and only one specifically mentioned the systems approach for problem solving and organizing for service delivery.

Parts of many individual responses were positive and indeed provided a sound basis for debate during the conference and for the images of the future that have developed since. It is certain that many participants, given a second look at their responses and those of fellow members, would have found them incomplete and would have spotted inadequacies. Yet these responses seem to reflect problems and conflicts among those trying to do school health and also point the way to specific areas where progress is not only possible, but also readily achievable.

THE FUTURE OF SCHOOL HEALTH

In the time since the conference, a number of positive images have taken form. If some of our shortcomings were revealed in the images exercise, more of our latent strengths were to come forth in the interaction that followed. In the following pages we discuss some of these images, both those we feel *will* be a part of our future, and those we believe *ought* to be.

Image No. 1: School Health—Alive and Well

It comes as no surprise that there continues to be some anxious concern over the future health of school health. Although no one at the conference or in the field working every day is complacent about the struggles ahead, it is clearer today than every before that if school health did not exist, we would have to invent it. The problems are there; the children are there—or, better still, the need is there with a way of meeting it.

No one claims that the task is not complex. Education and health care have long existed side-by-side as two basic institutions of our society, with relatively little effective interaction and only sporadic cooperation. Long-established patterns of service delivery have kept both institutions functioning in traditional isolation, often operating as though they were hermetically sealed chambers. As a consequence, a tacit agreement has been reached to ignore the fact that the clientele of these two systems (particularly the children and adolescents) have been identical. Many of us have arrived at the conclusion that what has really been ignored is the growing child in his family. By placing three interrelated institutions— schools, health care, and families—into the context of the total community, we will identify the arena within which we are *in fact* operating, whether we choose to recognize it or not.

The traditional perspective each of us brings from our own institution or system (education or health) requires us to view most outside issues as "problems to be solved" or as "obstacles to be overcome" so our own system can continue to move smoothly toward its established goals. By stepping outside of our "skin" and seeing the larger whole, we are able to see where we, too, might be a "problem" for another system. Walter Kelly's Pogo said, "We have met the enemy, and he is us."

Even many of the problems we face are, in fact, indications of the unique opportunities of school health. The gap between the education and health care systems or the abrasions where they overlap—this is precisely where the children and their families are to be found. They do not fit into categorical slots, and their resistance to cubbyholing creates problems for us. But these are our problems, not theirs.

Quibbling over who should do what can become just that rare opportunity for professionals to work together across disciplines. If the health and educational systems do not understand each other and how to work together, that is exactly where our task is—to create the intersystem arrangements to make it possible to do excellent school health. Where else is it possible to have access to all the children, assessing health status and identifying needs? What other activity provides the means of smoothing access of health care for children who need it? And where else is it possible to go beyond passive referral and take on active roles: home visiting when necessary, brokering services for children, and even engaging in advocacy when the need arises?

Under what other auspices outside the school, would it be possible to foster the new generation of innovative health education? Where else can children be influenced through curriculum, but even more through trained teachers, to learn life skills, concepts of wellness, and responsibility for health leading toward disease prevention and health maintenance?

There is no doubt that school health is alive and well. This image is vivid and should stay with us. If some of us have difficulty believing in its future because of what we see it doing, we must affirm that future nevertheless, simply because the need is so great.

Image No. 2: The People in School Health

The people who are active in school health present an outstanding image. Any organization or program is based first of all on its people—who they are, and how they feel about themselves and their work and about the future of their activity.[3] For this reason, the conference focused on the people in school health, attempting to establish an environment in which we were all encouraged to step outside our professional roles, take off the badges, and make an effort to communicate with each other.

By all counts, it worked. The people took the conference format and expanded upon it, involving themselves enthusiastically in the planned activities as well as in the social occasions. A frequently repeated remark was, "The most important thing about the conference for me has been the people whom I have met and talked with far into the night."

A wide variety of people were present, with many disciplines and localities represented, as can be seen from the participant list in the Appendix. They were knowledgeable, forward-looking, and willing to share. As one person who had been in the field for a long time remarked, "Where did all of these bright, energetic, restless people come from? The quality of people involved in school health greatly encourages me for the future."

Fittingly, the idea of people as a basic resource[4] seemed to take hold at the conference. At the end, one administrator said, "I realize that I have overlooked a major resource on my own doorstep—*my staff*. I've got to get home and develop *my* people." Also not insignificant is the number of people who came from great distances, many at considerable sacrifice. As long as any endeavor has people with potential who have faith in its worth and future, it has a high probability of success.

Image No. 3: School Health as Interdisciplinary

To speak of school health as interdisciplinary is like saying the "school health of school health." It is not only interdisciplinary by definition, in that it bridges two systems, but its interdiscplinary nature is embedded in its name: *school* plus *health*.

The interdisciplinary team is a catchword in the literature and among professionals in many fields. It was no less so at the conference. Strong efforts were made to step outside our "professional skins," and no one was really surprised to find it still difficult—and hard to listen. From sources throughout the conference, we picked up comments similar to one participant's, when she said, "Watching the community teams, I realized that I don't remember a time in our schools in which people representing all those different areas sat down to work on a problem."

As to the difficulty in listening to efforts to communicate across disciplines (let alone work toward a common outcome) in some of the Task Force groups at the conference, another participant was moved to remark: "As a total outsider, I often felt like I was drowning in the jargon, caught between the moving fault lines of this collection of professionals who are out to define (or is it justify?) whatever it is that they do (or might do) in schools to improve the health of children." And yet a third, ruefully recognizing that we have often paid lip service to an ideal that we too seldom practice, stated, "We always get together in our own professional groups to talk about problems, when most of our problems are with *other groups*. But it's so hard to listen!"

Yet, the *problem* of communicating provides exactly that *opportunity* for professionals from different disciplines to work together, to accomplish ends that neither can handle alone. Much has been written about those gains that can result from teaching,[5] though many have found it to be a far from happy experience in practice. The synergistic gains, however, could be likened to the difference between viewing a scene through a monochromatic lens and then having the lens removed, seeing the scene in full vivid color and all dimensions. Seen from the perspective of one color, one does not even realize the lack of perception. The multiple view of situations available to an interdisciplinary team allows all of them to be aware of and act upon aspects of the problem that no single member could have fully recognized.

It is not surprising that incipient pessimism remains concerning the validity of interdisciplinary activity. Therefore, it is of utmost importance to identify what is actually going on when there is conflict. When there is a problem, a conflict, it is *people* who are in conflict. It is not a system or a discipline that is to blame—systems are people. These are problems of intergroup conflict that require people skills to manage and overcome.[6]

These skills do, in fact, exist in the study of facilitating group behavior, introduced to most of us at one time or another as group dynamics.[7] We may know something about intergroup conflict, but too often we do not have the skills to manage it.

There is ample experience in school health to state unequivocally that there is no interdisciplinry problem that is inherently insoluble. Every conflict is potentially negotiable. When it seems not to be, look to the people involved, not the problem, or to their discipline or system membership. Experience has abundantly demonstrated that when people are willing to make a commitment to common goals *and, therefore, to solve all problems,* they will find a way to do so.[8] "Where there is a will, there is a way," but never forget that the skills and understanding of group process are essential, even when the people are well intentioned.

Out of the activity of the conference and from many other sources, we can assert that there is no need for pessimism concerning the possibility of sound interdisciplinary interaction in school health. It is possible to negotiate workable arrangements between the professionals in each system. On the larger scene, the health care system *is* accepting redefined roles for professionals, and the educational system *does* show reform on many points.[9] And beyond that, everything school health does moves toward goals of either the health or the educational systems. Nothing in the goals or purposes of school health are inimical or contradictory to the goals of either system.

Finally, an exuberant comment of a participant at the close of the conference seemed particularly *apropos*. He said:

"Inter"- "multi"- or "omni"- disciplinary ... we worked *together* here across boundaries that not only included school and health people, but the community as well. We've got to have more opportunity to involve administrative and elected types in workshops. School health of necessity involves an amazing cross section of a community's functioning institutions.

Image No. 4: School Health and Expanding Participation

An attractive image that is emerging for school health in the future is that participation of students, parents, and the larger community is expanding. Participation implies not only a way in which activities and programs may be carried out, but also a philosophical stance.[10]

The literature of applied behavioral science is full of the value of participation for those who participate. Lee Carey[11] speaks of the development of human competencies, the interpersonal skills, and even the interpsychic development that takes place when people actively participate in the decisions and structures that affect their lives. Similar results are reported in the literature of social work, group dynamics, and adult education.

Student participation in school health has become an attractive idea. With increasing dialogue on the rights and responsibility of children, new roles for them in their own health care and education are being taken seriously. Both education and health are exploring ways of moving students out of passive "acted-upon" roles into active "doer" roles. Screening and inoculation programs require little involvement by the student. Involving the student in an individualized set of health goals, based on a personalized health profile, takes a little more initiative.

Many ways of "activiating" children's particpation have been suggested. One interesting example concerns utilizing the development of a particular program in school health for a school district as an opportunity for participation. A little imagination can find ways to engage student participation at many levels.

1. Work out exercises for getting small children's input, ideas, images, and attitudes on the issue.
2. Bring elementary children in an organized way to early committee meetings as the problem is studied, having them take turns as committee members during selected discussion.
3. Conduct classroom exercises on planning the health program or identifying the health problem, with adult committee members in attendance. Plan it well to raise children's interest in the program so they will look forward to the results.

4. Have children prepare and present a panel to adult groups, the committee, or professionals.
5. Organize students to do a survey on themselves (with expert assistance), suggesting a means of solving health behavior-related problems.
6. Design an exercise to clarify values for junior high or older elementary groups.
7. Develop a schoolwide committee in high school sociology or health classes to perform a major data-gathering project that would lead to participatory planning with administrators and school board members.

There is no doubt that it is far easier to think up examples than to carry them out. We must become very sure of ourselves and our belief in the value of participation to endure the difficulties. Participatory programs are conceptually untidy and often noisy, less efficient, difficult to control, and harder to evaluate by conventional means.[12] Beyond these problems, however, it is incredibly difficult to "deprofessionalize" an area of former professional control and expertise and to tolerate apparently less effective program activities on the part of nonprofessional participants. You really have to *believe*.

The arena of parental participation in school health is broader. As with most professional systems, our attitude toward laymen—parents in this case—is ambivalent at best. Participation on their part often means doing what we have designated as best for them and their children. If we are truly able to open up more avenues of authentic participation for parents, it will have a salutary effect on our health and education systems. It is a sobering reflection that we must overcome generations of consistent discouragement by health and educational systems of any real lay interest or involvement in the workings of these systems. Laymen often tend to view health care as glacially condescending and education as an impenetrable bureaucracy. Anything we can do to change the images we all have of each other is of extreme importance to us all. Just how important is developed in the following image.

Image No. 5: School Health and the Community

In a familiar statement, one of the participants summed up the prevailing attitude of many toward the community when she said, "The community—we've got to educate the community about school health." The fact that this is entirely true does not save it from also being entirely "ethnocentric." An equally accurate and perhaps more important statement would be that the community needs to educate school health about the community.

The image of school health in the future will depend in large measure on how well it learns about the community. There are signs that school health has, in fact, become conscious of that larger system. One indication of this is the growing use of outreach workers to establish communication with high risk and hard to reach populations.[13] By developing and elaborating on this effort to respond to the complex needs and characteristics of the community, school health will be saying that it is really ready to do whatever it takes to meet the health needs of children and their families.

A great image for school health in the future will come to fact when the health of children becomes a community issue. There are those who believe that some of the stubborn barriers to excellent school health can be surmounted only by active participation and support from the larger community. Major policy decisions on adequate funding, for example, or decisions to integrate health into the total curriculum, or any other innovative change will be possible only when community support has been developed beforehand. It really is essential that the historical tendency of health and educational professionals to discourage participation by the community be overcome and reversed.

Finally, community participation in the planning is imperative if plans are to reflect the needs of the community adequately. Far too often, planning for both health and education has been isolated from the community as a whole. Intelligent and expert planning efforts have produced unworkable programs that were out of step with the community, whereas efforts that began with the people instead of the problem have produced plans that reflect in their very fabric the unique characteristics of the community.[14] But this, as all forms of participation, is clumsy and often offends the professionals' desires for neatness and efficiency. It is hard to calculate how much might rest on our learning to tolerate, and even embrace, the participation of the community.

When the term, "Options for School Health," was introduced, it was a long time before anyone asked, "whose options?" It should be clear by now that these are the communities' options. School health itself is an expression of the communities' concern for the health of its children and families.

Image No. 6: Exploration of the Possibilities in School Health

One senses in many conversations that school health could be on the brink of a fertile period of exploration and experiment. If a breakthrough can be achieved in organizational designs to fit specific community profiles, with adequate funding to keep a good staff for sufficient time periods, a number of fascinating research projects might be possible in the near future.

Everyone is really interested in *what works*. What are the optimum ways of doing school health in various settings? How can cost-effective programs be developed that will show demonstrable changes in the health status of children? How can the more innovative health education programs be evaluated? What can truly influence health attitudes and behavior for children and their families?

A small but significant example illustrated some of the points outlined above. Following the conference, one participant, Jerry Kindred, sent back some comments including the following:

> I would like to focus more on what has been or is being done for kids. The conference dealt more with roles than needs and programs (things that work or don't work). For example, the *New York Times,* in its spring education issue, reported that in New York City, third-graders studying science at Community School 152 in the Bronx learn about the circulatory system through acting and movement. "Dana Manno, an actress and choreographer working as an artist in residence, has taught children to *act out* parts of the body. Four students form themselves into a living heart, with a child on a drum acting as the pacemaker, student drops of blood are pulsed through the heart as valves open and close. Other children form the lung, draped with streamers for arteries and veins and balloons for alveola." Is that a good program? Does it fit the existing fabric of health education? What were the strategies used to get the program into operation? How is it evaluated?

Kindred went on to say that school health people must break their second-class citizen status by ending their policy of piggybacking or plugging in to existing programs. If they are to be effective, they must plan and evolve with the leading edge of the educational reform movement that is moving on many fronts.

The question remains as to how the necessary cross-fertilization can be facilitated and how the developing new knowledge can be adequately communicated to all of us in school health. If synergy is to occur, there must be sustained interaction.

Image No. 7: School Health Doing a New Thing—Planning for Change

The final image for the future of school health is perhaps the most significant of them all, yet there is no guarantee that it will become an image of the future, nor indeed is there anything like a consensus that it should. The one element almost totally missing from the "Images of the Future" exercise concerned how to organize and plan for change in social systems. As mentioned earlier, only one person among the more than 200 in attendance referred to this directly as a needed image of the future.

By the time the conference closed, however, many were agreeing with one participant who explained, "It all comes down to *change*. Good grief, how much longer can we run away from that?"

This was exactly what we observed in the Community Studies sessions. What was more significant than the specific problems they solved was that they had managed to bring about change. Many viewed these examples with caution, yet with some rising hope. The questions that began to hover in the air were, "Can we really do such a thing? Are there really ways to make it happen?" It is also most significant that pessimism occurred mostly during the workshop sessions on "barriers." The mood of some that afternoon seemed to be that "It's out of our hands, what can we do?"

After a decade of experience, more is now coming forth in the literature concerning the new technology of organizational development and systems change. There are numerous models, the principles of which are readily available.[15] The detailed development of a community plan for change in school health is the proper subject of another monograph. What is most significant here is to open up this image as a real possibility for the future.

Although not all may agree, little is "new" in school health since the basic goals were laid down by the World Health Organization (WHO) over 25 years ago. The health needs in children are clear, and the technology has long existed. The focus, then, must shift and concentrate on *how* we do it, rather than remain arrested at the "what do we do?" stage. We must define goals that transcend the familar ones in our respective bailiwicks and develop specific objectives for action toward those goals. We must develop a basis for interaction between the systems, not just an *interface*. We must see our activity as joint action and ourselves as mutual components of a larger system—the human community. From this perspective, the whole can become significantly greater than the sum of its parts. Synergy becomes a possibility. The new thing in school health becomes how to structure it; that is, how to utilize the new technology of organization change and development.

If we adhere to these goals for change, it is possible to identify some of the "hows": how to identify change processes in our respective systems and harness them to this issue, how to create new intersystem organizational structures to realize the possibilities of school health to meet the needs of children in our communities, and how to identify and focus the necessary resources in our respective systems to make it all possible.

Are we ready to deal with the fact that the status quo does not exist in any human social system? Are we ready to admit that perhaps it is a comfortable myth that allows us to decry the lack of change without having to take the risks of participating in change?

All social systems are constantly undergoing change. Processes that bring about change are constant, ongoing, and can be identified in any social system.[16] *Goal-directed intervention in those ongoing change processes is possible and can be planned.*[17]

This is a challenge to many of our casually held assumptions about organizations, bureaucracies, and other types of social systems. And what of the community itself? All of our activities exist as components (or subsystems) of that larger system, the community. What role should other systems in the community play in the future of school health? These questions must be considered in looking at any specific strategies for developing school health programs in the future.

System concepts are widely used and probably just as widely abused. The value of using a systems approach to talk about organization is that it allows change, growth, and development, while giving a perspective that can deal with the complexities of social systems. Because it is dynamic, it depicts change as continuous and enables us to talk about change in terms of process.

The usefulness of this approach is apparent in that it finally frees us from trying to create *the model* for school health, or coming up with *the definition.* Our search for a blueprint or a structure, as though school health were an institution, is over. Options for school health can really begin to make sense. School health is simply a practical intersystem arrangement, the focus for a cluster of well-understood activities with defined objectives and desirable outcomes.

The question remains, should this approach be one of the images of the future of school health, perhaps *the* image? More to the point, should school health people learn to bring about change?

In Proverbs, the writer observed that "Where there is no vision, the people perish." The vision of our possible future becomes the most critical of all of our activities.

Summary: The Images in Retrospect

Nothing is more sure than change in any system. We are all aware of the slow pace with which change may occur in our various systems. But change processes are always underway in all social systems. The slower the process, the more energy is being expended to maintain that slow pace. There is no such thing as a static system. Either we take the initiative and focus the changes in our various social systems toward desirable goals, or we will continue to be passive spectators of change processes we have not planned, do not want, and are helpless to prevent. Or worse still, we may be unwilling participants in change processes running counter to our best instincts and our professional judgments. Who has not experienced that familiar frustration? It is not hard to understand why the myths of intransigent bureaucracies have developed, as we find ourselves apparently helpless to influence the seemingly inevitable course of large bureaucratic organizations.

But bureaucracies are organizations, and that means people—people acting in groups. The dynamics of people in groups have been studied. Organizations can be understood and can be changed. Knowledge of how this can happen is available to all of us.

As long as we allow ourselves to believe that things are somehow "out of our hands" and that there is no way to bring about change, we will continue in our role of observers and recorders carefully measuring effects that we did not cause, scientifically describing phenomena that powerfully influence people's lives but remaining helpless to do anything about it. Then we will continue to talk about "objectivity" and "professional distance" and the "ethics of intervention," using these and other concepts to protect us from the stark facts of human misery and our inability or unwillingness to act. After all this comes our failure of nerve.

There is, then, a possible image for the future of school health in which key people have developed the requisite skills in planning, group process, community participation, and system change. In that image we see options for school health being exactly those appropriate for the community and effectively responding to the health needs of our children and their families.

CONCLUSION

Reflections on School Health: The State of the Art

In the two years since the National School Health Conference, developments have been followed in the various communities that came to the conference, and feedback from individual participants has been gathered as well. The accumulated experience, together with recent developments, seems to indicate that the time was ripe for exploring options in school health. The objectives of that conference can be restated simply: to develop a workable theoretical structure for school health; to outline specific objectives and guidelines for school health; to identify basic methods for implementing school health programs in a variety of settings; and to test the validity of the objectives, guidelines, and methods against the concrete experience of living communities. Several things have occurred toward these objectives. In reverse order: we have had the opportunity to test the validity of many of the objectives, guidelines, and methods against the concrete experience of living communities. Although more testing and research will be necessary, some methods have been identified to implement school health in a variety of settings, and experience continues to accumulate on the specific objectives and guidelines for school health that are now being tested in many places.

It is with the first objective (one of structure and definition) that the most concrete progress may have been achieved, and that progress is to eliminate it altogether as a meaningful objective. We may be rid of our persistent longing for "the structure," or "the model," or at least "the definition" for school health that would solve our problems and provide us with a foolproof blueprint and an established methodology. Nowhere in any of the materials in preparation for the National School Health Conference, nor in this book, is there an attempt to present the final definition of school health. Although "what is school health?" is still one of the most frequently asked questions, it has finally become clear that to think of school health in terms of concrete definitions leads all thinking in the wrong direction.

School health is not a single, distinct entity, which somehow continues to elude all of our efforts at definition and defies our attempts at categorization. School health is a systems term, a convenient short phrase referring to a cluster of related activities whereby the community attempts to improve the health of children and their families through planned programs requiring cooperative action of the educational and health caring systems. This means that the initiative to identify the specific needs of a given community, and to plan programs to meet those needs, lies precisely *in that community*. What we now see emerging is collaboration by the professionals in the educational and health care systems to develop carefully designed joint actions, tailored to those needs, with the details developed through active participation of students, parents, and the larger community.

Professionals in both the educational and health caring systems have an absolutely essential set of new tasks to perform to realize the promise of school health. Some among us must become skilled in the new technology of planning and organizational change in complex social systems.

While providing the expertise to develop the necessary intersystem arrangements to do school health, these professionals must also recover or retrain themselves in the long-neglected group skills needed to help complex human groups become synergistic. We must set examples of openness, tolerance, and accepting behavior in our cross-disciplinary endeavors, making it possible for people from a variety of factions in the community to meet one another as persons first of all and then to discover ways to work toward the common goal of improving the health of our children and their families. Persons with professional roles in both health and education must move out of determining absolutely the goals and objectives of school health for a given community and move into roles of facilitating, developing, enabling, consulting, and providing necessary expertise. Most of all, these parties must act as partners with the community, sharing responsibility as well as knowledge, receiving as well as giving guidance. This is a very difficult challenge, but the experiences of those who are moving in this direction indicate that the rewards are worth the effort.

School health, then, as an organized arrangement or intersystem activity, does not "belong" to either the health or educational system as such (although in a given community one or the other may take the lead responsibility in developing it). It belongs to the community, as do both the health and educational systems in the final analysis; it is the community's way of getting at a variety of health needs of children and their families. School health is not a new and competing service system, nor a developing discipline, nor even a profession. It is not the "answer" to all problems in a given community concerning either the health or the education of children. It is rather a concrete, practical problem-solving activity, a useful arrangement for meeting health needs, and most of all, a process that allows for all who participate—professionals, parents, students, and community persons—to come forth with the best possible solution to the problem addressed. Finally, school health, in this understanding, will be able to be continuously responsive to changes and developments in the needs of children and their families and will be open to modification or elaboration as the community requires.

These are the images of school health that are important for our present and immediate future. And if we do our work well, new images will be developed by this process.

REFERENCES

1. Analysis of the "Imaging the Future" exercise sheets that were handed in that first day, coupled with the results of the conference itself, provided the concept and the materials for this final chapter.

2. This has been noted in many meetings of professionals, especially where a high percentage of those in attendance are involved in direct service delivery or in first level supervision. Those involved in consultation with business and industry have also indicated that this is frequently the case. See R. Beckhard, *Organization Development: Strategies and Models* (Reading, Mass.: Addison-Wesley, 1969).

3. Numerous works in modern management theory are pointing out that this is essential. An excellent example is D. McGregor, *The Human Side of Enterprise* (New York: McGraw-Hill, 1960).

4. Pursuing this idea in extensive field research with many organizations is the comprehensive report, R. Likert, *The Human Organization: Its Management and Value* (New York: McGraw-Hill, 1967).

5. The listing of articles having to do with the value and methods of interdiscipline is not possible in this space. Nursing and education have been long in this field, with medicine joining more recently (and some think more reluctantly). The basis for any learning effort, however, is simply laid out in E.H. Schein, *Process Consultation: Its Role in Organization Development* (Reading, Mass.: Addison-Wesley, 1969).

6. As good a place to begin is with Beckhard, *op. cit.* The problems associated with change in social systems are also well covered in the basic text for change agents: W. G. Bennis, K. D. Benne, and R. Chin, *The Planning of Change* (New York: Holt, Rinehart and Winston, 1969).

7. One starting point is with K. Benne and P. Sheals, "Functional Roles of Group Members," *Journal of Social Issues* 2, (1968), as outlined in Schein, *op. cit.* Much of the research is found in the work of D. Cartwright and A. Zander, Eds., *Group Dynamics: Research and Theory* (New York: Harper and Row, 1960).

8. A fundamental premise of group dynamics. See Reference 7.

9. As has been illustrated by the previous chapters in this book. See specifically Chapters 3 and 4.

10. The literature on the values and effects of citizen participation has focused primarily on those who have traditionally been excluded from participation. The concept is, however, only a modern assertion of a traditional value and as such is needed in most areas of our society. See E. M. Burke, "Citizen Participation Strategies," *Journal of the American Institute of Planners* 34, no. 5 (Sept. 1968).

11. Lee J. Carey, Ed., *Community Development as Process* (Columbus, Mo.: University of Missouri, 1970).

12. A point that many have used to resist the utilization of the participatory approach to planning and change. See H. Goldblatt, "Arguments For and Against Citizen Participation," in *Citizen Participation in Urban Development,* Vol. 1, H. B. C. Spiegel, Ed. (Washington, D. C.: National Institute for Applied Behavioral Sciences, 1968).

13. Although this is a relatively new area, there is abundant evidence that it can be a most effective means of establishing a new kind of relationship between the professionals of service delivery systems and the client population whom they are attempting to serve, i.e., the community. For example, see C. Dorrofrio, "Aides, Pain or Panacea," *Public Health*

Reports 85, no. 9 (Sept. 1970); G. Hildenbrand, "Guidelines for Effective Use of Non-professionals," *Public Health Reports* 85, no. 9 (Sept. 1970); and R. Reiff and F. Reissman, *The Indigenous Nonprofessional* (National Institute of Labor, 1977).

14. For a more detailed discussion of community planning as applied to health services, see J. G. Bruhn and J. A. Williams, "Community Planning for Emergency Medical Services," in *First Aid in Emergency Care*, G. Parcel, Ed. (St. Louis, Mo.: C.V. Mosby, 1977).

15. Look at R. Chin and K. Benne, "General Strategies for Effecting Change in Human Systems," in *The Planning of Change and Organization for Social Change: Action Principles from Social Science Research*, Bennis *et al.*, Eds. (New York: Columbia University Press, 1964); and the venerable but still highly valuable work of M. G. Ross, *Case Histories in Community Organization* (New York: Harper Brothers, 1958). For yet another perspective on how human organizations function, see E. H. Schein, *Organizational Psychology* (Englewood Cliffs, N.J.: Prentice-Hall, 1970).

16. Recent thinking about social systems has been liberated from the homeostatic conceptualizations of Talcott Parsons. This has resulted in many fertile ideas that give new insight into how human groups and organizations interact. One of the most stimulating is the work of W. Buckley, "Society as a Complex Adaptive System," in *Modern Systems Research for Behaviorial Scientists*, W. Buckley, Ed. (Chicago: The Aldine Company, 1968). A more elaborate treatment, placed in its historical context, is Buckley's *Sociology and Modern Systems Theory* (Englewood Cliffs, N.J.: Prentice-Hall, 1967). Application of these principles is showing up in a variety of areas, such as G. Hearn, Ed., *The General Systems Approach: Contributing Toward an Holistic Conception of Social Work* (New York: Council on Social Work Education, 1969).

17. This statement contains the essence of the approaches outlined in this chapter. It is fundamental to any conceptualization of *planned change;* and it asserts that it is, in fact, possible to exercise some control on the future.

Appendix

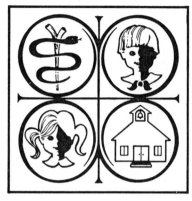

Options for School Health

CONFERENCE CONCEPTS AND OBJECTIVES

Objectives

The National School Health Conference was held in Galveston, Texas, at the end of the second year of a five-year demonstration and research project in comprehensive school health. The objectives for the conference were simply stated as:

1. to develop a workable theoretical structure for school health;
2. to outline specific objectives and guidelines for school health;
3. to identify basic methods for implementing school health programs in a variety of settings; and
4. to test the validity of the objectives, guidelines, and methods against the concrete experience of living communities.

The admittedly ambitious objectives of the conference, the positive language of the preconference materials, and the long and careful preparation led to a number of participants almost triple the 70 to 75 originally envisioned and planned for by the steering committee. How all this came about is the subject of this Appendix.

Concepts

Traditionally, most conferences are called for the purpose of getting professional people together who are working in common areas with the hope of exchanging information and stimulating new directions. New developments in a field of endeavor are usually presented in a formal way, either from a theoretical or historical perspective. Practical experience can, on occasion, be presented in workshops or case studies. People come, listen, pick up copies of the presented papers, and go home.

The National School Health Conference proposed to go beyond the familiar format of conferences of this type. The objectives of the conference were ambitious and required that we plan an atypical task-oriented conference format. We brought many capable people together from a broad spectrum of backgrounds, including professionals in health and education, laymen, other professionals with related expertise and high interest, and the emerging community-oriented paraprofessional roles in health and education. To realize fully the potential contributions of those who attended, we needed to create a participatory learning environment that was open, experimental, and developmental. In this setting we hoped not only to learn from the planned presentations but also from each other by actively engaging in dialogue and problem solving. It is in this way that the conference worked toward accomplishing its objectives.

Therefore, in addition to doing the usual things that conferences attempt to do, we wanted to try for a further step—to make a little history as well. We hoped to create an experimental learning environment where theory could be developed further and steps could be taken in its application in a real, live community. We hoped not only to report on working school health programs, but also to participate in starting new ones based on the best we know and on the shared experiences of the participants who attended the conference.

PRECONFERENCE PROCESS

From the outset, planning for the National School Health Conference had two basic characteristics: (1) the idea, "options for school health," emerged out of a recognized need to help schools and communities organize, change, or expand their school health programs; in other words, the germ for what became the Community Studies existed at the beginning; and (2) the informal group that became the steering committee was an *interdisciplinary* team.

As the group began to examine the ideas that were to become the objectives for the conference, it became obvious that the format must be participatory, people focused, and task oriented. This led to the decision to make this a relatively small invitational conference, hopefully of 70 or so persons from around the country who were active in school health, knowledgeable of its problems and promise, and representing a cross section of disciplines currently involved in school health.

As the concept of examining options developed, it was decided to request position papers on current issues in school health from among those to be invited. These papers were to be both theoretical and practical in nature, looking at models as well as ideas and objectives. It was envisioned that this collection of papers, modified and expanded by the interaction resulting from the conference, would form the material for a monograph on options for school health. Those papers did become, in fact, the basis for the chapters in this book.

As the steering committee contained several people with long experience in school health, the first round of invitations was sent to a selected cross-section of school health people across the country. Included in the invitation was a request to identify any others who might make a contribution to a conference of this type. There was also a request for comments or suggestions.

At this point the avalanche began. Enthusiastic responses listed many others. Some replies came in, copied from someone else's invitation, asking to be allowed to attend. When the participant list had to be closed due to limitations of staff and space, over 200 people were confirmed as coming to the conference.

The steering committee had developed a program that included a balance between presenting information in the form of addresses, panels, etc., and group participation activities, such as task forces and workshops (see conference program schedule in this Appendix). The sharp increase in the number of participants put a severe stress on developing adequate participation opportunities, in that maintaining small group sizes and providing capable staffing are both essential to the success of this format.

Probably the most significant events of this preconference period centered around the development of the Community Study concept as a major conference activity and the time spent with each of the community teams assisting them to prepare their presentation. The concept evolved to become that of a "living case study" to be presented as a half-day workshop at the conference and timed to focus the conference participants on real situations for their problem-solving exercises. This would prevent the rest of the conference activity— which included theory building, Task Force activity, problem-solving exercises, and working models— from becoming ends in themselves, presented for the enlightenment or at least entertainment of those attending the conference. Rather, these were to become events in a process aimed at concrete action. Options for school health were to be developed by the participants as they worked together at the conference, and steps toward application of these options in the three Texas communities were to have begun before everyone left the conference site.

Selecting the communities for the Community Study sessions proved to be amazingly easy. The steering committee reviewed a number of communities that would present a variety of settings, demographics, and types of school systems. Various problems in availability of and accessibility to health care were also a consideration. The schools of the three communities of Hidalgo, Odessa, and Austin were approached; and all three readily agreed to develop a Community Study session for the conference. They quickly assembled a group representing the schools and health services in the community and got busy.

Working with the three community teams as they prepared for the conference was itself a study in options for school health. A member of the steering committee took on the role of liaison for each Community Study team, making several visits during the months prior to the conference. Several of the steering committee members were able to travel to the cities, both to encourage the teams and to help their own learning. All began to sense that something important was happening.

During this time the committee developed a Guideline for Community Study to assist the team in their preparation. This document itself, although designed for this specific purpose, is also a helpful model for initiating other planning for school health.

As the number of conference participants grew, the steering committee became seriously concerned about the fact that only three community study sessions could not possibly accommodate such large groups and still maintain a participatory workshop format. Just as the committee began to think of trying to reach out for another community, a group of participants from the Boston area and the Harvard School of Public Health requested to be allowed to bring a team from a nearby community with which they were familiar. That is the way that Worcester, Massachusetts, became the fourth Community Study session, adding greatly to the interest and variety of the conference, as well as providing another, very different community to study.

SETTING THE STAGE

One of the assumptions of the conference steering committee was that people in school health need to have opportunity to get outside their "professional skin" and meet each other as persons outside the confines of professional or discipline boundaries. The stage for the conference was set so people could "take off their badges" and try working together toward common goals in school health.

It is an interesting paradox that the more open and participatory an event is to become, the more care is required in planning. As an additional challenge the conference staff took on the presumptuous and always risky task of trying to do some role modeling in climate-setting and creating the kind of learning environment where the conference objectives could be achieved. Some of the climate-setting activities included: (1) volunteers meeting and greeting people at the airport with their cars to reduce the hassle of getting to the conference site; (2) a message center that not only kept messages but actively assisted participants in looking each other up; (3) a core of hostesses to provide assistance in working out all kinds of little problems; (4) a smooth registration procedure; (5) daily publication of a conference newsletter to provide cohesion, with instructions, information, and comments from participants; (6) detailed conference packets, with extra copies of materials for those who needed them; (7) preregistration list and a daily update of all participants (see final list in this Appendix); and (8) informal social gatherings, such as a barbecue and wine and cheese parties, planned to provide additional unstructured settings for people to meet and interact. Perhaps the most important thing, however, was the attitude of the conference staff and all who helped make the event possible. The people set the climate in any setting, and this conference was no exception.

THE CONFERENCE

First Night

Carrying forward the standards of the conference, the opening event was a social hour followed by dinner. Name tags had *names only,* no credentials. All had been informed that no ties would be allowed. There was no head table and no formal greetings by dignitaries (this necessary formality was saved until the first session on the following morning). Staff circulated, meeting and introducing people to each other.

After dinner, a brief climate-setting exercise led to the first event of the conference, the convening of the Task Force groups. These groups were to be the "home group" for the participants and would meet periodically throughout the conference, working together on specific tasks. Therefore, the members had been carefully preselected and assigned to create a heterogeneous blend of people in each group. The members of the various Community Study teams were dispersed so every Task Force had some of these individuals in it. Other types of participants such as the new paraprofessionals and outreach workers were similarly dispersed. Each group had cofacilitators as staff.

At the end of the first evening, which was devoted to group-building and the sharing of expectations, the conference staff was remarking on the high level of knowledge, talent, interest, concern, and enthusiasm they found in their groups. By the end of the next day, the participants themselves were beginning to realize the same thing. In other words, they began to feel good about the quality of people in school health.

First Day

The opening session began with an exercise in "Imaging the Future." This provided many insights into the group, which are discussed in some detail in Chapter 7. Suffice it to say now, perhaps the most outstanding result of this initial exercise was that the participants began to realize, as a group, that they did not know what success looked like, nor did they know how to identify the kinds of goals necessary for effective planning.

The morning session progressed through the scheduled address and panel, communicating considerable information, ideas, theories, and, in the discussions that followed, opinions on school health. After lunch the first Task Force session took place, revealing some additional things about the participants. Here members of the four Community Study teams, scattered as they were among five Task Force groups, had the opportunity to engage with other participants in a problem-solving task. This was one of the occasions where the steering committee had hoped that getting a wide variety of people together as a common task would have a synergetic effect. Furthermore, the plan and Program Guideline for the afternoon task force session provided a problem-solving model that could be used by interdisciplinary groups as they worked on problems in school health.

The outcomes of the Task Force workshop were difficult to assess. During the reporting session it was clear that many had found the barriers almost overwhelming. Although some groups had come out with some specific strategies to achieve the objectives for school health that were under examination, most had not been able to get far beyond the problems into possible solutions. It was clear that the barriers for many seemed insurmountable, that resources seemed woefully inadequate, and that most participants needed to know more about what can work to feel that success was possible.

In the Task Force activity it first began to be obvious that, as a group, the participants were lacking in basic planning skills and that many of them had no knowledge of how to go about effecting change in complex social systems; nor did they seem to have much faith that such change is possible. The need of the group for skills in the new technology of organizational change was beginning to surface.

During the afternoon, the planned interaction of interdisciplinary Task Force groups was a rare experience for many participants. A number commented on how refreshing it was to do, but how hard it was to listen to, as people stumbled against each other's jargon.

The evening concluded with an informal barbeque event, which eased the tensions of many participants. For some, the close of the first day marked the end of their inflated expectations and the beginning of realism. For others, the all too familiar pessimism began to return.

Second Day

Opening the second full day of the conference was an unscheduled event of some significance. On the previous evening, word had come to the conference coordinator that a group of participants who worked as community workers, aides, home-school agents, and outreach workers were very unhappy about the content and direction of many of the Task Force groups and were considering leaving the conference. Acting quickly, he gathered about nine of them together to discuss the reason for their unhappiness. It should be mentioned here that in preparation for the conference, this group had been briefed and told that they should attempt, whenever possible, to represent the concerns of the families they saw daily in their work and, to the degree possible, the interests of the large community outside the health and educational system. All of these individuals were women, were from minority groups, and were indigenous to the low and moderate income areas of their respective communities.

The group agreed to meet with the coordinator and to share with him their frustrations. One person summed it up fairly well:

> It's not just the jargon, although that's pretty bad. It's that some of us don't feel that anyone is even interested in what we have to contribute about families—even though they all talk about "involving the families" as though it's some magic word. Every time I try to open my mouth, someone interrupts to talk about trying for some grant under some Title I to X. You would think these folks didn't live in the world, to hear them talk.

As discussion progressed, it became clear that participants in the conference had been making the familiar mistake of plunging deeply into professional dialogue, which took them further and further from the real world where outreach workers lived daily. And if they did not have the patience and the courtesy to listen to fellow conference members, asked one aide, what were they doing in their own activities at home?— a question worth posing. Another pointed out that all her group had talked about was roles and how they should relate to each other. She wondered if they would ever get around to relating to the community.

After some discussion, the conference coordinator asked the group to repeat this discussion, just as it had taken place, before the whole conference the following morning. Fearful and trembling, they consented. They were not at all sure it would help, but they were willing to give it a try.

Therefore, when the conference participants assembled on the morning of the second day, the large room had been rearranged. All chairs were arranged "in the round," leaving a small ring of chairs in the center. In this ring were the community workers, frozen stiff with fright. After a brief introduction, explaining the event and the fishbowl technique, in which the group would try to continue the discussion began the evening before, the conference coordinator sat down in the circle and started the group off. It was tough going for a few minutes until they got warmed up. Finally, out of anger as much as fright, several repeated their observation of the evening before. With encouragement from the coordinator, others joined in until the picture of their frustration was clear to all the conference participants. As the coordinator brought the session to an end after only ten minutes, the silence was profound in the room. The coordinator thanked the community workers warmly for their concern, and particularly for their courage, and proceeded without further comment into the scheduled program for the day. Later in the day, one of the outreach workers observed that she could hardly cough without someone asking her to repeat her remark.

The flow of information continued during the morning of the second day. An address and a dual panel explored some concrete models of school health programs that were relatively successful. The participants were eager to hear more. All this led up to the afternoon of the second day, which was scheduled for the Community Study sessions.

Community Study Sessions

Many of the members of the various Community Study teams had become deeply involved in the conference. Some of them admitted to a real wrench when they realized that they were about to become a part of the program. By now, they were aware that they were a key part of the conference.

The specific content of each Community Study session is discussed in Chapter 5. It is sufficient here to outline how the sessions were structured and how they were received by the other conference participants.

A guideline for the Community Study sessions was prepared for the members of the team and one for the facilitators of the session. These form an interesting model for a participatory workshop on community problems in school health and are included in this Appendix.

The introduction to the Community Study sessions focused on the community to a degree not yet seen at the conference. The plan for the sessions included a community profile, thus making it clear that school health programs, as well as the health and educational systems, exist in a larger system, that is, the *community*. There is no way to avoid this reality.

Setting the stage for the Community Study sessions was important. An explanation of the afternoon's activity was presented to the assembled participants before they broke up to attend the various sessions. In it, they were told that their role was as consultants, sitting in with the community team. These teams were actively working on a specific problem in school health in their community and were having this week's meeting at the conference. They had identified a problem on which they needed to work, and the participants in each session were being invited to consult with them on possible steps in solving the problem. The responsibility for the problem was to rest with the teams. It was a *real* problem, and they would continue to live with their solution after they returned to their communities.

The Community Study sessions were set up to give conference participants the opportunity to test the various objectives, guidelines, and methods that had been discussed in the conference sessions thus far. By having to deal with the concrete experiences of living communities in a workshop setting, the participants would have an opportunity to help develop strategies for action that were based on reality. At the same time, the community teams would have the benefit of the broad range of expertise and experience of the other participants as they worked together.

The four Community Study sessions were presented simultaneously on Tuesday afternoon, the second day, from 1:40 to 5:00 p.m. with an additional hour on the following morning for wrap-up. Conference participants were assigned to the separate sessions, according to preference. The assignments were made in such a way to ensure that each group had a variety of members representing different disciplines, and that the Task Force groups were scattered among all four Community Study sessions. It appeared that each Community Study session had between 20 and 30 participants present in addition to the community team members and the liaison person.

Under the guidance of the team leader and the liaison person, the community team presented the pertinent information on their community and schools, outlined the current status of school health, and offered a specific problem for the participants in the Community Study session to work on during the afternoon. The problem represented the next step needed for further development of an adequate school health program in that particular community. The outcomes of the session would be a plan for a blueprint for a feasible program to solve the problem presented by the community team. The detailed accounting of what occurred in each community team session is found in Chapter 5.

Thursday—Closure

The Community Study sessions reconvened Thursday morning and completed the details of their work. Then the Task Force groups reconvened and tried to make some sense of it all, sharing the impressions that the various members of each Task Force had obtained from the different Community Study sessions. Finally, the conference gathered restlessly for a closing summary.

It would be difficult to describe the complex mood of the conference at its close. Clearly an altering of expectations had occurred, but with little loss of enthusiasm. If anything, the group was more intense, arguing to the last. They realized that they had come as knowledgeable, yet somewhat naive, individuals from a variety of settings. Some were in the know concerning contemporary issues in school health, while others had been more isolated. They were together in school health but in many ways were separated by the real difficulties of interdisciplinary communication. They had received no "final answers," nor had they found the definitive definition of school health. Certainly they had not produced the "theoretical structure" of school health as stated in the conference objectives; but that seemed to matter very little, even though it had been the first objective of the conference. They had tested the many objectives, guidelines, and methods suggested at the conference against some living communities, and the results seemed to be both sobering and stimulating.

Many showed impatience with the searching, reaching, and struggling type of language (i.e., groping) and expressed their desire to become more intentional, to use building, constructing, and synthesizing images. There was a sense that the group was perhaps just now ready to get specific, to look at *what works,* to consider research and evaluation of creative programs. In the closing discussion, there was also a decided shift toward health education, which had often become lost in the shuffle during the conference.

The conference evaluation forms filled out by the participants were fascinating. Almost uniformly positive, they were characterized by detailed lists of things to do when the participants returned home. Many described specific insights that they were carrying away. Although there seemed to be a reluctance to leave, there was clearly an impatience to get on with it. There was throughout the evaluations a clear call for communication, for mutual support, for help, for knowledge, for skill. Finally, many had experienced the feeling that school health was not in such bad shape, that they could see it moving into its future, exploring its options.

THE FOLLOW-UP

The National School Health Conference was designed to develop a theoretical framework for school health and to identify strategies for implementing school health programs in various types of communities. The task-oriented conference brought together a broad spectrum of professionals and laymen interested in school health. Four communities were invited to participate as case studies. Community representatives presented the current state of school health in their communities. All conference attendees participated in problem solving in the Community Study sessions.

An immediate postconference follow-up asked participants to state their goals and objectives for school health for the following year. The stated goals and objectives were used as a basis for a questionnaire mailed to participants nine months after the conference. The areas of involvement dealt with in the questionnaire included: (1) sharing information; (2) roles and role reorientation; (3) education and training; and (4) organization. In addition, the participants were asked to identify barriers to school health that they had found during the past year and to comment on how they dealt with these barriers. In a concluding section respondents identified the type of aid they would need to achieve their school health goals. Of the 179 questionnaires sent out, 113 (63 percent) replied with a sufficient amount of information to be tabluated. Those who responded were a cross-section of those who attended the conference; that is, all professional disciplines were represented.

Sharing Information

Of the respondents stating that they had been actively involved in sharing information concerning school health, the great majority shared information concerning the conference with colleagues. In addition, 14 of the respondents were involved in evaluation of school health programs.

Services

The majority of the respondents were involved in screening programs or providing services for children involved in special education programs. One conference participant had worked out an emergency alert system and medical priority rating system for special education students. Another was involved in developing health programs for day care children.

Roles and Role Reorientation

Involvement by participants in developing roles in school health included expanding the role of the school nurse, adding paraprofessional workers, and the development of the team approach to school health. In developing new roles, the conference participants were involved in a variety of ways. These included: (1) using the pediatric nurse practitioner as a school nurse; (2) having the nurse practitioner provide primary care in the schools; and (3) training health advocates in day care settings. Some respondents indicated health aides were added to schools. In one setting, rural health care was expanded by the hiring of a school nurse.

Education and Training

Establishing and expanding health education programs appeared to have been another primary focus of the respondents' work during the year following the conference. Many participants indicated that they were involved in developing health education programs within schools or for parents. Some were developing educational experiences for professionals involved in school health.

The development of continuing education experiences for the nurses and health teams was an area of emphasis for the conference participants. In addition, many provided training experiences for health science students of all types. Parent in-service and educational programs were designed to encompass the areas of general health, child health, and child abuse. New health education programs focused in the high school on parenting skills and in grades three and four on health and safety.

Organization

Many respondents said they had been busy establishing goals for their school health programs and furthering contacts between community health care resources and schools. Several individuals found it worthwhile to establish a community advisory council on school health and/or to conduct a survey of existing resources in the community. One participant noted the reactivation of a community advisory council on school health. A directory of services available to students was developed by one district. Contacts were established through conference with health care providers, parent advisory groups, and one-to-one meetings.

Barriers to Achievement of School Health Goals

Participants were asked to select from a list of nine potential barriers to school health, the ones that they felt were most impeding their objectives. They were also asked to explain how they dealt with the barriers they found. The barriers encountered varied greatly; however, many people noted a lack of time and funds to pursue their objectives. Personal contact was the primary method specified to deal with the barriers of lack of information and lack of communication within the health system and the community. Indeed, direct contact with personnel, doctors, clinics, and parents seems to be one method many participants used to overcome barriers to their school health objectives. Conferences, inservices, and workshops also accomplish much of the same purpose as direct contact. In regard to the barrier of community attitudes toward school health, one conference participant noted that, "Health in most communities doesn't seem to the number one priority." An explanation of why there is a lack of information by school officials concerning school health was given: "Since most schools never had a health program, they don't know what it is."

One nurse involved in working in a school health room stated that, "Not enough time allowed to work health problems in two schools, due to: (1) clerical work requiring duplication of forms; and (2) a large enrollment of students requiring a full-time nurse to care for health problems."

One respondent found a solution to the problem of lack of funds by working with the department of social services and using early and periodic screening funds by billing Medicaid directly for services rendered. In this program, the school nurse provided direct primary care to the school population. Poor coordination among regulatory agencies was another barrier found during the year following the conference by many conference participants.

Needed Assistance

The respondents were asked what type of assistance they felt they would need to achieve their desired school health programs. The four categories were: staff, finances, administrative coordinator, and consultation services. A great number of people felt the need for consultation services in many areas. These ranged from developing new services, roles, and programs to determining the needs of the population, to influencing school administrators to view the health programs with a higher priority. The areas in which people felt they needed consultation most were developing new health education programs and determining the needs of the population. It is postulated that this may, in fact, reflect the two areas that respondents were least involved in during the year following the conference.

ANNOUNCING: A National School Health Conference

OPTIONS FOR SCHOOL HEALTH

June 20-23, 1976   Galveston, Texas

SPONSORED BY:

The Robert Wood Johnson Foundation

CO-SPONSORED BY:

Galveston Independent School District
Catholic Schools of Galveston-Houston
The University of Texas System School of Nursing at Galveston
The University of Texas Medical Branch at Galveston

School Health Services—Today's Challenge

Expectations and responsibilities of the public and private schools in
the area of health care for children continue to expand at an accelerating
pace. Schools across the land have always found themselves in contact
with children for a greater part of their waking hours during 12 significant years of their lives. Although still important, those traditional
school health activities— such as proper handling of sick children during
school hours (including emergencies) and the familiar routine screening
and health education programs— are no longer capable of meeting the increasing new demands.

The long-established right to education, upon which democracy is
based, is now recognized to be inextricably linked to the emerging "right
to health" for every citizen. The children in our communities with
unresolved health problems and without adequate knowledge or ability
in their families to maintain wellness cannot develop their full potential
in the education system. They are therefore blocked from full participation in the whole life of this society. We are now coming to a recognition
of these facts and beginning to realize the social, emotional, and financial
costs to us all.

Change—The Most Challenging Problem

Education and health care— these two basic institutions of our society
have long existed side-by-side with relatively little effective interaction
and only sporadic cooperation. Long-established patterns of service

delivery have often kept both institutions functioning in traditional isolation so that they frequently operate as though they were in hermetically sealed chambers. This has resulted in the tacit agreement to ignore the fact that, particulary with children and adolescents, the clientele of these two systems has been identical. Many of us have arrived at the conclusion that what has really been ignored as a result is that other even more basic institution in our society—the growing child in his family. By placing three interrelated institutions—schools, health care, and families—into context of the total community, we can begin to identify the arena within which we are *in fact* operating, whether we choose to recognize it or not.

The traditional perspective which each of us has from within our own institutions or systems (education or health) requires us to view most things from outside our respective systems as "problems to be solved" or as "obstacles to be overcome" in order for our own system to continue to move smoothly toward its established goals. By stepping outside of our "skin," so to speak, and seeing the larger whole, we are able to see where we, too, may have been a "problem" for another system—in other words, we have all been part of the problem as often as part of the solution. Perhaps we are beginning to understand the profound simplicity of Walter Kelly's Pogo, when he said "We have met the enemy, and he is us."

Doing a New Thing—Planning for Change

As most of us are aware, there is little that is actually "new" in school health since the basic goals were laid down by the World Health Organization (WHO) over 25 years ago. The health needs in children are clear, and the technology has long existed. The focus, then, must shift and concentrate on *how* we do it, rather than remain arrested at the "what do we do?" stage. In other words, we are saying nothing less than it has become necessary to recognize the need for superordinate goals which transcend our familiar system goals in our respective traditional bailiwicks and to develop specific objectives for action to those goals. We must develop a basis for intersystem *interaction,* not just *"interface."* We must see our activity as joint action and ourselves as mutual components of a larger system, the human community. From this perspective, the whole can become significantly greater than the sum of its parts. Synergy becomes a possibility. The *new* thing in school becomes *how* to structure it, i.e., how to utilize the new technology of organization change and development.

Change goals of this type make is possible to begin identifying some of the *hows:*

- how to identify change processes in our respective systems and harness them to this issue;
- how to create new intersystem organizational structures to realize the possibilities of school health to meet the needs of children in our communities;
- how to identify and focus the necessary resources in our respective systems to make it all possible.

From *this* perspective, the *resources* of our communities can be seen in an entirely different light— not as severely limited commodities for which there is already too great a competition, but as essentially unlimited potential, already present in the strengths of the individuals, families, reference groups, and institutions of the whole community and of the society in which we live. Our greatest danger will not be in planning too big, but with our timid reflexes in *thinking too small!*

Conference Objectives

The accumulated experience of the health and educational system, together with recent developments, indicates that the time is ripe for exploring options in school health. Old problems and new challenges will require new steps if the promise of school health is to be realized. In this context, the objectives of this conference can be simply stated as:

1. to develop a workable theoretical structure for school health;
2. to outline specific objectives and guidelines for school health;
3. to identify basic methods for implementing school health programs in a variety of settings; and
4. to test the validity of the objectives, guidelines, and methods against the concrete experience of living communities.

The Program

Traditionally, conferences are called for the purpose of getting people together who are working in common areas with the hope of exchanging information and stimulating new directions. New developments in a field of endeavor are usually dealt with in a formal way, either from a theoretical or historical perspective. Practical experience may on occasion be presented in workshops or case studies.

The National Conference on School Health proposes to go beyond the familiar format of conferences of this type. The objectives of the conference are admittedly ambitious and have required that we plan an atypical task-oriented conference format. We are bringing many capable people together from a broad spectrum of backgrounds, including professionals in health and education, laymen and other professionals with related expertise and high interest, and the emerging community-oriented roles in health and education. To realize fully the potential contributions of those who will attend, we need to create a participatory learning environment that is open, experimental, and developmental. In this setting we cannot only learn from the planned presentations but also from each other by actively engaging in dialogue and problem-solving. It is in this way that the conference can accomplish its objectives.

Therefore, in addition to doing the usual things which conferences attempt to do, we want to try for a further step—*to make a little history as well*. We hope to create an experimental learning environment where theory can be developed further, and steps can be taken toward its application in a real, live community. We hope not only to report on working school health programs, but to participate in starting new ones based on the best we know and on the shared experiences of the participants who attend the conference.

With this end in mind, we are inviting several communities and cities in Texas to send teams composed of key persons representing health care, the educational system, and the community itself. These teams will be prepared to be "living" case studies. The teams will present the current state of school health in their respective communities. They and the conference participants will work together on these problems in the Community Study sessions. It is here that we will test the validity of the objectives and methods that we develop against the concrete experience of these communities. All who attend the conference will have the opportunity to participate in one of the problem-solving case studies.

Conference Schedule

The purpose of this schedule is to show the overall structure and flow of the conference, which is the result of months of planning. While many of the speakers and panelists have been identified and will be announced soon, the ultimate success of the conference will depend on the all-important *process*. The focus at this point is on *how* these planned events are to be carried out, and how those who attend will be able to participate.

Sunday, June 20

5:00 p.m.	Registration
6:30 p.m.	Reception/cocktails
7:30 p.m.	Dinner

8:30 p.m.	Presentation: Ideas and Concepts of the National School Health Conference—Climate Setting for the Conference
8:50 p.m.	Formation of Task Groups for the Conference
9:00 p.m.	Group Building Session—Open Ended

Monday, June 21

8:30 a.m.	Convene—Introduction and Climate Setting
8:40 a.m.	Mini-groups: Brainstorm "Image of the Future"
9:10 a.m.	Welcome
9:30 a.m.	Address
	Questions and Answers
10:15 a.m.	Coffee
10:30 a.m.	Panel
11:30 a.m.	Discussion
12:15 p.m.	Lunch Break
1:30 p.m.	Task Forces Groups: Convene and Accept Tasks
1:45 p.m.	Task Force Group Action
4:00 p.m.	Panel: Task Force Group Leaders
	Discussion
5:00 p.m.	Adjourn

Tuesday, June 22

8:30 a.m.	Convene—Introduction and Climate Setting
8:40 a.m.	Address
9:15 a.m.	Discussion
9:45 a.m.	Coffee
10:00 a.m.	Models of School Health: Panel—Cambridge, Massachusetts, School Health Program and Galveston, Texas, School Health Program
	Questions and Answers
12:00 p.m.	Lunch Break
1:30 p.m.	Community Study Sessions
5:00 p.m.	Adjourn
Evening	Social to be Announced

Wednesday, June 23

8:30 a.m.	Convene—Update and Climate Setting
8:40 a.m.	Community Studies (continued)
10:45 a.m.	Coffee
11:00 a.m.	The Future of School Health: Summary and Discussion
11:45 a.m.	Closing Remarks
Noon	Adjourn

Preparation

Preconference materials are currently under preparation for those who will participate in the conference. While we expect to keep preparation on the part of participants to within manageable limits, some thought and reading will be valuable to have us all ready to work when the conference convenes.

At the conference, the historical analysis, the theory building, the Task Force activity, the working models, and Community Studies will not be ends in themselves, presented for the enlightenment or at least entertainment of the conference attendees. Rather, these will become events in a process aimed toward concrete action. Options for School Health will be developed by the participants as we work together at the conference, and steps toward application of these options in the three Texas communities will have begun before we leave the conference site.

Everyone who participates should be amply warned that they have come to share their knowledge and experience and to learn new things—not by passively receiving information but by active involvement in problem solving.

The new dimension which we will strive to develop as we gather is ACTION.

The University of Texas Medical Branch at Galveston
January 1976

NATIONAL SCHOOL HEALTH CONFERENCE
OPTIONS FOR SCHOOL HEALTH

Guidelines for Task Force Groups

The National School Health Conference is designed to work toward developing a theoretical framework for school health and to identify strategies for implementing school health programs in various types of communities.

The conference proposes to go beyond the familiar format of conferences of this type. The objectives of the conference are admittedly ambitious and have required that we plan an atypical task-oriented conference format. We are bringing many capable people together from a broad spectrum of backgrounds, including professionals in health and education, laymen and other professionals with related expertise and high interest, and the emerging community-oriented roles in health and education. To realize fully the potential contributions of those who will attend, we need to create a participatory learning environment that is open, experimental, and developmental. In this setting we cannot only learn from the planned presentations but also from each other by actively engaging in dialogue and problem solving. It is in this way that the conference can accomplish its objectives.

The Task Force groups are a key activity in establishing the necessary learning environment for the conference. The groups form an important arena where the heterogenous participants can interact and learn from each other. They are also the major opportunity for the knowledge and experience of the participants to be fed into the conference itself.

Specifically, the Task Force groups at the National School Health Conference have been set up with the following purposes in mind:

1. to provide a "home group" to meet several times during the conference and help give continuity. The participants will be able to meet and interact with each other in the nonformal setting, becoming comfortable enough to work together;
2. to increase the opportunity for participation by individuals and to provide a place to explore, test out, and to challenge the ideas presented by panels and speakers;
3. to create a working group which can tackle the specific tasks related to the Objectives of School Health, thereby making their knowledge and experience available to each other and giving them the opportunity to have input into the results of the whole conference; and
4. to integrate the conference experience for the group members, discussing and coming to some conclusions on the conference objec-

tives (i.e., the Task Forces will be the place where work on the conference objectives will be most facilitated).

The Task Force groups are scheduled to meet simultaneously three times during the conference: (1) Sunday night, for a relatively brief but open-ended session to develop the group and to establish expectations; (2) Monday afternoon for four hours to work on an assigned task; and (3) Wednesday morning, to achieve some integration of the conference experience.

Conference participants will be assigned to the Task Force groups to ensure a heterogenous mix of professions and geographic areas. Each group will be staffed by a team of two cofacilitators and a research assistant. Specific tasks will be presented to the groups for workshop sessions on Monday afternoon. It will be up to the participants, however, to make the Task Force groups into a useful activity. The teams of facilitators can assist in keeping a focus during the sessions and offering suggestions on ways to work on the tasks.

If the group members engage with each other offering concrete examples from the vast experience represented here at the conference, the purposes of the Task Force groups have a chance of being fulfilled. Try to maintain a level of discussion somewhat less global than "all children have a right to health" and a little more general than a discussion on how to write Title I grants. In other words, focus on the organizational and systems level—the place where achieving the "Objectives for School Health" will in fact be worked out.

Finally, most everyone has had some experience in groups. Any group can prevent the special interest of an individual or a small group from dominating it or sidetracking it from its essential purposes. Don't allow this to happen. In other words, *the Task Force groups need to take responsibility for their own productivity.*

NATIONAL SCHOOL HEALTH CONFERENCE
OPTIONS FOR SCHOOL HEALTH

Introduction: Community Study Sessions

The National School Health Conference is designed to work toward developing a theoretical framework for school health, and to identify strategies for implementing school health programs in various types of communities.

The Community Study sessions are set up to give conference participants the opportunity to test the various objectives, guidelines, and methods which have been discussed in the conference sessions thus far.* By having to deal with the concrete experiences of living communities in a workshop setting, the participants will be able to develop strategies for action that are based in reality. At the same time, the community teams will have the benefit of the broad range of expertise and experience as the participants work with them on the problems to be solved.

The four Community Study sessions will be presented simultaneously on Tuesday afternoon, June 22, from 1:40 to 5:00 p.m., with an additional hour for wrap-up on the following morning. Conference participants will be assigned to the separate sessions, according to preference and to ensure an adequate number in each session. It appears that each Community Study session may have between 30 and 40 participants present in addition to the community team members and the liaison person.

Under the guidance of the team leader, the liaison person, and/or group facilitator, the community team will present the pertinent information on their community and schools, outline the current status of school health, and offer a specific problem for the Community Study session to work on during the afternoon. The problem should represent the next step needed for further development of an adequate school health program in that particular community. The outcome of the session will be a plan or blueprint for a feasible program to solve the problem presented by the community team.

Procedure

This guideline is offered to assist the community team in preparing and focusing their presentation and to help participants understand their role in the Community Study sessions.

---

* See Conference Schedule.

The Community Study sessions are planned to proceed as follows:

1. Presentation of the community and the problems to be worked on
   a. Distribution of profile data package (before Community Study session)
   b. Introduction of Community Study team members and the community-liaison person
   c. Slide presentation: community team
   d. Summary of the status of school health in the community: community team
   e. Presentation of the problem to be worked on: community team
   f. Questions and answers for clarification only

   -break-

2. Workshop activity: conference participants and community team members working together on the problem, using modified "fishbowl" technique
3. Closure: decisions or options for solution to problem and plans for action. Agreement on a sequence of steps to solve the problem

As can be seen from the simple outline above, once the community team members present their community with the specific problem to be studied, they will work together with the participants for the remainder of the time available. The whole group is responsible for the outcomes. Whatever results from the Community Study session depends on the participation of everyone present.

NATIONAL SCHOOL HEALTH CONFERENCE
OPTIONS FOR SCHOOL HEALTH

Working Notes: Community Study Sessions

Introduction

The National School Health Conference is designed to develop a theoretical framework for school health and to identify strategies for implementing school health programs in various types of communities.

There is a need to bring together people from around the country who have experience and/or expertise in developing new approaches to school health. There is also a growing group of educational and health care personnel interested in developing or enhancing their community school health and child health care programs. If successful, the conference can create an atmosphere and a task orientation which will make it possible to achieve the objectives of the conference, which are:

1. to develop a workable theoretical structure for school health;
2. to outline specific objectives and guidelines for school health;
3. to identify basic methods for implementing school health programs in a variety of settings.

Purpose of Community Study Sessions

In order to achieve the objectives listed above, it is necessary to add a fourth objective, which is:

4. to test the validity of the objectives, guidelines, and methods against the concrete experience of living communities.

It is to achieve this fourth objective that the Community Study sessions are included in the conference format. Several communities in Texas are being asked to send community teams to the conference, prepared to take a lead role in the Community Study sessions. These communities have been selected to represent a broad spectrum of sizes, settings, histories, demographic configurations, and resources available for school health activities. The one common characteristic of the teams is their interest in working on the problems and challenges of school health in their own community.

The Community Study sessions will be set up to give the conference participants the challenge of testing the validity of what they have been doing in the conference thus far, by wrestling with the application of theory to real community problems. By working in small groups with the community teams, the participants will have the experience of developing strategies for action, while the community team members will have the benefit of a broad range of participants working with them in the small groups. The Community Study sessions will be given focus by experienced group leaders, who will assist the team members and participants in the problems to be worked and achieve some closure in the time available.

Preparation

Community teams will consist of five to seven (or more, if indicated) people from the schools, the health care providers, and the community at large. The individuals to comprise the team are selected because of their key roles in the decision-making structure of the community and for their interest in school health and child health care. They will be prepared to present the salient facts of the school health problems from their own community (which they have selected for the Community Study sessions to work on) and will participate in these sessions with conference attendees in working toward developing solutions to these problems.

Preparations on the part of the community teams will be necessary. Conference staff will visit the communities and assist in orienting the team members for the Community Study sessions. One conference staff member will be identified as the liaison person and will assist the community in putting together a brief but comprehensive description of their community, the schools, and the health care system. In this community setting, the teams will present the selected problems in school health to work on during the Community Study sessions. No two communities will be the same, so the work of conference staff with the community team in the months prior to the conference becomes very important.

The community studies will be kept relatively uncomplicated in order for the problem-solving function of the sessions to be achieved. The most effective way of presenting each community profile and the specific school health problems to be worked on will be determined in the preconference meeting with the team members and the conference staff. These could include some or all of the following:

1. printed profile data on the community and the schools;
2. maps and charts;
3. brief presentation by some community team members;
4. slides on the community, if available;
5. other visuals as needed.

More detailed guidelines for gathering information for community profiles and for making the community studies presentation will be developed with each community team by the conference staff.

The University of Texas Medical Branch at Galveston
January 1976

Community Study Sessions

Tuesday: Working Session. After the presentation of community and the problem to be worked is complete, explain procedure for working session—the modified "fishbowl" technique.

Group Tasks	*Facilitator Tasks*
1. Team members, with consultants restate the problem into an objective that can be reached (i.e., what are we trying to do? what is our target?).	1. Bring four to five participants to table as "consultants" and begin discussion on objective.
2. Reach agreement on objective through a brief discussion.	2. Write on wall chart the objective agreed upon.
3. Team moves to consider the specific steps that must be taken to reach the objective.	3. With consultants, identify steps. (May find "back chaining" a useful tool; may break group in two groups, etc.).
4. Arrange the steps into a logical sequence of events.	4. Write steps on prepared wall charts. Arrange in sequence.
5. Examine: What will it take to do each step? What changes or actions are needed? What coordination, what resources?	5. Write changes/actions/coordinations on chart. Write resources/costs on charts.
6. Team members alone make final decision on each step and on the actions necessary. Forced closure by end of session on each step.	6. Consultants, entire team comes to closure on each step, final decision is team's alone.

Wednesday Morning: Convene with community team only at table.

---

1. Review the sequence of steps and the actions necessary. Make any adjustments.

2. General discussion: make a list of alternatives, exceptions, or "minority report" items on a chart for team to have.

3. Dismiss to Task Force groups.

1. Team alone goes over steps briefly.

2. Open to floor. General discussion, getting in ideas, alternatives not accepted by team—listing on chart; also, "minority report" type of comments.

Newsprint charts on walls.

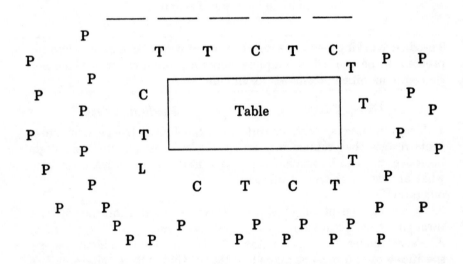

P=Participants   L=Liaison Person

T=Team members   C="Consultants"

Product of the Community Study session: a "plan" or blueprint, so to speak. Specifically, a sequence of steps to take that will achieve the objective that the Community Study team decides on—i.e., a "solution" to the problem with necessary changes or actions identified (key coordination activities in particular) and required resources indicated.

NATIONAL SCHOOL HEALTH CONFERENCE
STEERING COMMITTEE

Philip R. Nader, M.D.
Conference Coordinator
Associate Professor of Pediatrics and
    Psychiatry and Behavioral Sciences
Director, School Health Programs
University of Texas Medical Branch

John G. Bruhn, Ph.D.
Associate Dean of Medicine
Coordinator of Community Affairs
Professor of Preventive Medicine & Community Health
University of Texas Medical Branch

Elizabeth Fitzsimmons
Administrative Assistant to
    Executive Dean of Medicine
University of Texas Medical Branch

Rosemary McKevitt, R.N., Ed.D.
Formerly: Nurse Educator and Consultant
School Health Programs
University of Texas Medical Branch
Present: University of Texas School of Nursing
    at San Antonio, Texas

Guy S. Parcel, Ph.D.
Assistant Professor of Pediatrics and
    Preventive Medicine and Community Health
Health Educator, School Health Programs
University of Texas Medical Branch

James Williams, M.S.W.
Coordinator for Educational Planning
Office of Dean of Medicine
University of Texas Medical Branch

Mildred Williamson, R.N.
Coordinator of Health Services
Galveston Independent School District

TASK FORCE GROUP LEADERS

Alan Appelbaum
Victor Azios
Ernest Barratt
Pat Blakeney
Dorothy Bullock
Bill Caldwell
Edna Courville

Rosalind Berrey
Bonnie Canavan
Sandra Carey
Lupita Castilleja

Facilitators

Lucy Guzman
Rosemary McKevitt
Alice Anne O'Donell
Diane Roberts
Richard Smith
Barbara Williams
Gregg Wright

Recorders

Michael Meyer
Peggy Stanley
Kathy Tiernan

PARTICIPANTS IN NATIONAL SCHOOL HEALTH CONFERENCE — OPTIONS FOR SCHOOL HEALTH

Alabama

Martha D. Adams
Supervisor of School Nurses
Birmingham Public Schools
Birmingham, Alabama 35203

California

Robert J. Meeker
Psychology Department
University of California at Los Angeles
Manhattan Beach, California 90266

Jerold C. Kindred
Shelter Institute
149 Ninth Street
San Francisco, California 94103

Colorado

K. Victoria Hertel
School Nursing Consultant
Colorado Department of Health
Denver, Colorado 80220

Patricia A. Motz
School Nurse Practitioner
Chairperson
American Nurses' Association Ad Hoc Committee on School Health
Denver Public Schools
Denver, Colorado 80231

Helen Ridge
Supervisor of Nursing
Denver Public Schools
Denver, Colorado 80224

Connecticut

Judy Lewis
Instructor
Model School Health Project Director
Department of Pediatrics
University of Connecticut Health Center
Farmington, Connecticut 06032

Margaretta E. Patterson
Assistant Professor of Pediatrics
University Community Health Center
Farmington, Connecticut 06032

District of Columbia

Gwen Bates
School Health Consultatnt
HEW
Washington, D.C. 20203

Florida

Rudy Maxwell
Manager, Agricultural Labor Project
Auburndale, Florida 33832

Georgia

Roy L. Davis
Director, Community Program Development
PHS-DCD Bureau of Health Education
Atlanta, Georgia

Illinois

Pauline Carlyon
Project Coordinator
National PTA
700 North Rush Street
Chicago, Illinois 60611

William Carlyon
Assistant Director Health Education
American Medical Association
535 North Dearborn Street
Chicago, Illinois 60611

Roger J. Meyer
Assistant Dean of Continuing Education
University of Illinois School of Public Health
2035 West Taylor
Chicago, Illinois 60612

Chieko Onoda
Pediatric Instructor
University of Illinois, College of Nursing
845 South Damen
Chicago, Illinois 60611

Marcia Opp
Bureau Chief, *Medical World News*
645 North Michigan
Chicago, Illinois 60611

William M. Young
President, Urban Dynamics
Oak Park, Illinois

Godfrey Cronin
Superintendent
Posen-Robbins School District
Posen, Illinois 60469

Indiana

Marjorie Ferguson
School Nurse Practitioner
School City of Gary
620 East 10th Place
Gary, Indiana 46407

Leanne Halfman
School Nurse Practitioner
School City of Gary
620 East 10th Place
Gary, Indiana 46407

Gordon McAndrew
Superintendent, Gary Schools
620 East 10th Place
Gary, Indiana 46407

Mary E. Young
School Nurse Practitioner
School City of Gary
620 East 10th Place
Gary, Indiana 46407

Kentucky

Faye Leverton
School Nurse Supervisor
Fayette County Health Department
330 Waller Avenue
Lexington, Kentucky 40504

Maryland

David Graham
Pediatrician—School Health Fellow
University of Maryland
5 Greene Street
Baltimore, Maryland 21207

Dolores Basco
Nurse Consultant
Division of Nursing, U.S. Public Health Service
Bethesda, Maryland 20014

A. Frederick North
President, Ambulatory Pediatric Association
Professor of Pediatrics & Public Health
University of Pittsburgh
Graduate School of Public Health
Bethesda, Maryland 20014

Katherine Kendall
Chief, Nursing Section
Bureau of Community Health Services
Department of HEW
5600 Fishers Lane
Rockville, Maryland 20852

Massachusetts

Robert Haggerty
Professor, Public Health and Pediatrics
Head, Health Services Administration and Maternal and Child Health
Harvard School of Public Health
677 Huntington Avenue
Boston, Massachusetts 02115

Katherine P. Messenger
Lecturer in Child Health
Harvard School of Public Health
677 Huntington Avenue
Boston, Massachusetts 02115

Judith S. Palfrey
Associate Director Community Service Program
Children's Hospital
333 Longwood Avenue
Boston, Massachusetts 02115

Kathryn West
Associate, Office of Extramural Health Programs
Harvard School of Public Health
677 Huntington Avenue
Boston, Massachusetts 02115

Leighton Davenport
Research Assistant
Cambridge Hospital
Cambridge, Massachusetts 02139

Judith A. Fellows
Public Health Analyst
Department of Health and Hospital
1493 Cambridge Street
Cambridge, Massachusetts 02139

Marilyn Germano
Public Health Assistant
Cambridge Hospital
Department of Pediatrics
Cambridge, Massachusetts 02139

Cynthia K. Gilbert
Nursing Supervisor
Department of Health and Hospital
1493 Cambridge Street
Cambridge, Massachusetts 02139

Philip J. Porter
Chief of Pediatrics
Cambridge Hospital
Cambridge, Massachusetts 02139

M. Lucinda Wilke
Pediatric Nurse Practitioner
Department of Health and Hospital
Cambridge, Massachusetts 02139

John R. Ford
Director, Human Services
City of Worcester
253 Belmont Street
Worcester, Massachusetts 01605

Margaret M. Hickey
Assistant Director of Public
   Health Nurses
Worcester Department of Health
19 Belmont Street
Worcester, Massachusetts 01605

Michael E. Huppert
Executive Director
Great Brook Valley Health Center
170 Tacoma Street
Worcester, Massachusetts 01605

Edna May Macewicz
Director, Public Health Nursing
Worcester Health Department
Worcester, Massachusetts 01605

John J. O'Neil
Director
Health, Physical Education &
   Safety
Worcester Public Schools
20 Irving Street
Worcester, Massachusetts 01609

John F. Smith
Director of Public Health
Worcester Department of Public
   Health
419 Belmont Street
Worcester, Massachusetts 01604

David E. St. John
Supervisor Pupil Personnel Ser-
   vices
Worcester Public School System
20 Irving Street
Worcester, Massachusetts 01609

James J. Underwood
Director of Special Education
Worcester Public School System
20 Irving Street
Worcester, Massachusetts 01609

Michigan

Roy E. Paterson
Vice President
Mott Children's Health Center
806 West Sixth Avenue
Flint, Michigan 48503

Minnesota

Ardyce Carlson
Administrative Supervisor Health
   Services
St. Paul Public Schools
360 Colborne
St. Paul, Minnesota 55106

Delphie Fredlund
Associate Professor, University of
   Minnesota
1325 Mayo
St. Paul-Minneapolis, Minnesota
   55455

New Jersey

Frank Jones
Program Officer
The Robert Wood Johnson Foun-
   dation
P.O. Box 2316
Princeton, New Jersey 08540

New York

Al Finkelstein
Director of Health Services
Community School District 18
1070 East 104 Street
Brooklyn, New York 11236

Susan Kaye
Assistant Director Special Services
Great Neck Public Schools
345 Lakeville Road
Great Neck, New York

Helen Schweser
Health Educator
Levittown, New York 11756

Loretta C. Ford
Dean and Director of Nursing
University of Rochester School of
  Nursing
601 Elmwood Avenue
Rochester, New York 14620

Stanley F. Novak
Director, School Health Programs
University of Rochester School of
  Medicine and Dentistry
260 Crittenden
Rochester, New York 14627

Richard E. Behrman
Professor and Chairman
Department of Pediatrics
Columbia University College of
  Physicians and Surgeons
New York, New York 10027

Philip Frieder
Department of Pediatrics
Columbia University College of
  Physicians and Surgeons
New York, New York 10027

Carroll F. Johnson
Professor of Educational Adminis-
  tration
Teachers College
Columbia University
New York, New York 10027

North Carolina

Michael R. Lawless
Assistant Professor of Pediatrics
Bowman Gray School of Medicine
Department of Pediatrics
Winston-Salem, North Carolina
  27103

Ohio

Isaac E. Hamilton
Supervisor—Division of Health
  and Family Life Education
Cleveland Board of Education
1380 East Sixth Street
Cleveland, Ohio 44122

Stephen J. Jerrick
Executive Director
American School Health Associ-
  ation
P.O. Box 238
Kent, Ohio 44240

Lillian F. Bernhagen
President, American School
  Health Association
(Former Director of Health Ser-
  vices, Worthington City Schools)
Worthington, Ohio 43085

Oklahoma

Orvella M. Hahn
School Nurse—Western Heights
School District
John Glenn School
6500 South Land
Oklahoma City, Oklahoma 73159

Nevin L. Starkey
Coordinator School Health Ser-
vices
Oklahoma State Department of
Health & Education
10th and Stonewall
Oklahoma City, Oklahoma 73117

Virginia Turvey
School Nurse
Director of Health Education
Board of Education
314 South Lewis
Stillwater, Oklahoma 74074

Pennsylvania

Annette Lynch
Director, Burned Children's Ser-
vices
Pennsylvania Department of
Health
Box 90
Harrisburg, Pennsylvania 17108

Foster H. Young, Jr.
Assistant Professor Community
Medicine
University of Pittsburgh Medical
School
Pittsburgh, Pennsylvania 15213

Jerold M. Aronson
Director, School Health Services
School District of Philadelphia
200 North 21st Street
Philadelphia, Pennsylvania 19103

Susan S. Aronson
Project Director, Health Advocacy
Training
The Medical College of Philadel-
phia
3300 Henry Avenue
Philadelphia, Pennsylvania 19129

Texas

Durward L. Bell
Director/Clinical Psychologist
Austin Child Guidance Center
Austin, Texas 78767

Charlene Bennett
School Nurse
Austin Independent School Dis-
trict
1216 Rio Grande
Austin, Texas 78731

Margaret R. Boice
Consultant
Texas Department Health
Resources
1100 West 49th Street
Austin, Texas 78756

P. A. Cato
Medical Advisor
Austin Independent School Dis-
trict
1701 Sylvan Drive
Austin, Texas 78741

James V. Clark
Director of Pupil Personnel Ser-
vices
Texas Education Agency
201 East 11th Street
Austin, Texas 78701

Herma E. Dawson
Administrator of Health Services
Austin Independent School District
1216 Rio Grande
Austin, Texas 78701

Lynn A. Frank
Chief Consultant, Texas Education Agency
201 East 11th Street
Austin, Texas 78701

Lillian M. Gilliam
Staff Development Specialist
Austin Independent School District
Austin, Texas 78767

Charlene Laramey
Administrative Assistant
Austin Independent School District
Austin, Texas 78752

Paula McCormick
Research Coordinator
Texas Department of Community Affairs
P.O. Box 13166, Capitol Station
Austin, Texas 78711

Mary Manning
Guidance, Visiting Teacher Consultant
Texas Education Agency
201 East 11th Street
Austin, Texas 78701

Janice M. Ozias
Supervisor of School Nurses
Austin Independent School District
6100 Guadalupe
Austin, Texas 78752

Gloria M. Pennington
Parent/Consumer
5607 Shoalcreek Blvd.
Austin, Texas 78756

P. Clift Price
Pediatrician
Texas Pediatric Society
School Physician, Texas School for Blind
Austin, Texas 78767

Wayne Rider
Principal
Austin Independent School District
6100 Guadalupe
Austin, Texas 78752

Reymundo Rodriguez
Executive Assistant
The Hogg Foundation for Mental Health
University of Texas at Austin
Austin, Texas 78712

Luisa Sanchez
Austin Independent School District
6101 Dillard Circle
Austin, Texas 78752

Helen H. Woods
Consulting School Physician
Corpus Christi Independent School District
Corpus Christi, Texas 78408

Percy Penn
Assistant Principal
Dallas Independent School District
3606 South Westmoreland
Dallas, Texas 75233

Adeline Anges
Pediatric Nurse Practitioner
Galveston Independent School District
Galveston, Texas 77750

Alan S. Appelbaum
Assistant Professor, Child Psychiatry
The University of Texas Medical Branch
Galveston, Texas 77750

Victor Azios
Social Worker
Galveston Independent School District
Galveston, Texas 77750

Jewel Banks
Principal
Galveston Independent School District
Galveston, Texas 77750

Ernest Barratt
Professor and Director
Behavioral Science Laboratory
The University of Texas Medical Branch
Galveston, Texas 77750

Rosalind T. Berrey
Research Technician, School Health Programs
The University of Texas Medical Branch
Galveston, Texas 77750

Robert K. Bing
Dean, School of Allied Health Sciences
The University of Texas Medical Branch
Galveston, Texas 77750

Pat Blakeney
Assistant Professor, Psychiatry
The University of Texas Medical Branch
Galveston, Texas 77750

Torik Bouhairie
Fellow, Ambulatory Pediatrics
The University of Texas Medical Branch
Galveston, Texas 77750

Larry E. Bradley
Instructor, Health Care Sciences
School of Allied Health Sciences
The University of Texas Medical Branch
Galveston, Texas 77550

John G. Bruhn
Associate Dean of Medicine
The University of Texas Medical Branch
Galveston, Texas 77550

Dorothy Bullock
Social Worker, Child Development Division
The University of Texas Medical Branch
Galveston, Texas 77550

Bill Caldwell
Associate Professor of Pediatrics
The University of Texas Medical Branch
Galveston, Texas 77550

Bonnie K. Canavan
Research Technician, School Health Programs
The University of Texas Medical Branch
Galveston, Texas 77550

Sandra Carey
Physician's Assistant Student
The University of Texas Medical
Branch
Galveston, Texas 77550

Lupita Castilleja
Student—Pan American University
Summer Internship
Galveston, Texas 77550

Effie Clark
School Nurse
Galveston Independent School
District
Galveston, Texas 77550

Jane Conrad
Pediatric Nurse Practitioner
Galveston Independent School
District
Galveston, Texas 77550

Edna Courville
Social Worker, Children & Youth
Project
The University of Texas Medical
Branch
Galveston, Texas 77550

C. W. Daeschner
Professor and Chairman
Department of Pediatrics
The University of Texas Medical
Branch
Galveston, Texas 77550

Sandra Dale
Instructor, School of Nursing
The University of Texas Medical
Branch
Galveston, Texas 77550

Dorothy M. Damewood
Dean, School of Nursing
The University of Texas
Medical Branch
Galveston, Texas 77550

Cassandra S. Deaver
Educational Consultant, School
Health Programs
The University of Texas Medical
Branch
Galveston, Texas 77550

Warren F. Dodge
Professor of Pediatrics
The University of Texas Medical
Branch
Galveston, Texas 77550

Gloria L. Ellisor
Pediatric Nurse Practitioner
Galveston Independent School
District
Galveston, Texas 77550

Leola Evans
Home-School Agent
Galveston Independent School
District
Galveston, Texas 77550

Chloe Floyd
Director of Continuing Education
School of Nursing
The University of Texas Medical
Branch
Galveston, Texas 77550

Velma Gordwin
Home-School Agent
Galveston Independent School
District
Galveston, Texas 77550

Don Gottlob
Director, Elementary Education
Galveston Independent School
District
Galveston, Texas 77550

Lucía Guzman
Assistant to the Dean
School of Allied Health Sciences
The University of Texas Medical
Branch
Galveston, Texas 77550

Barbara F. Johnson
Director, Division of Communications
The University of Texas Medical
Branch
Galveston, Texas 77550

Lois Jones
Coordinator of Home-School
Agents
Galveston Independent School
District
Galveston, Texas 77550

Edith K. Kelley
Director of Educational Development
School of Allied Health Sciences
The University of Texas Medical
Branch
Galveston, Texas 77550

Doris J. Kennedy
Home-School Agent
Galveston Independent School
District
Galveston, Texas 77550

Dolores Faye King
Pediatric Nurse Practitioner
Galveston Independent School
District
Galveston, Texas 77550

Tom Lasater
Principal
Galveston Independent School
District
Galveston, Texas 77550

Becky LeBus
Instructor, Occupational Therapy
School of Allied Health Sciences
The University of Texas Medical
Branch
Galveston, Texas 77550

Pat Lee
Social Worker, Early Childhood
Center
Galveston Independent School
District
Galveston, Texas 77550

Donna Livingston
Director of Special Services
Galveston Independent School
District
Galveston, Texas 77550

Rosemary K. McKevitt
Nurse Educator, School Health
Programs
The University of Texas Medical
Branch
Galveston, Texas 77550

A. W. Marchak
Director of Secondary Education
Galveston Independent School
District
Galveston, Texas 77550

Dorothy Marchak
Pediatric Nurse Practitioner
Galveston Independent School
District
Galveston, Texas 77550

Michael P. Meyer
Research Technician, School Health Programs
The University of Texas Medical Branch
Galveston, Texas 77550

Gerald E. Miltenberger
Director of Clinical Services
Center for Audiology & Speech Pathology
The University of Texas Medical Branch
Galveston, Texas 77550

Philip R. Nader
Director, School Health Programs
The University of Texas Medical Branch
Galveston, Texas 77550

Alice Anne O'Donell
Director, Family Medicine Resident Training
The University of Texas Medical Branch
Galveston, Texas 77550

Guy S. Parcel
Health Educator, School Health Programs
The University of Texas Medical Branch
Galveston, Texas 77550

Georgia A. Perrett
Pediatric Nurse Practitioner
Galveston Independent School District
Galveston, Texas 77550

Ernestine Prater
School Nurse
Galveston Independent School District
Galveston, Texas 77550

Vandell Price
Pediatric Nurse Practitioner
Galveston Independent School District
Galveston, Texas 77550

Marion K. Reinhart
School Nurse
Galveston Independent School District
Galveston, Texas 77550

Karen Riedel
Coordinator, Information Services
Galveston Independent School District
Galveston, Texas 77550

M. Diane Roberts
Chairman, Allied Health Services
School of Allied Health Sciences
The University of Texas Medical Branch
Galveston, Texas 77550

Sally Robinson
Pediatrician
Galveston, Texas 77550

Rose Mary Russell
School Nurse
Catholic Schools
Galveston, Texas 77550

Florence R. Sapio
School Nurse
Catholic Schools
Galveston, Texas 77550

Mary Frances Schottstaedt
Associate Professor of Psychiatry
The University of Texas Medical Branch
Galveston, Texas 77550

William Schottstaedt
Director, Area Health Education
  Center
The University of Texas Medical
  Branch
Galveston, Texas 77550

Mary Lou M. Shuffler
Social Worker
Galveston Independent School
  District
Galveston, Texas 77550

Richard D. Smith
Fellow, Behavioral Pediatrics
The University of Texas Medical
  Branch
Galveston, Texas 77550

Emma Dora Stanford
Home-School Agent
Galveston Independent School
  District
Galveston, Texas 77550

Peggy Stanley
Nurse
Galveston, Texas 77550

Kathy Tiernan
Research Technician, School
  Health Programs
The University of Texas Medical
  Branch
Galveston, Texas 77550

Patricia A. Toliver
Licensed Vocational Nurse,
  Children & Youth Project
The University of Texas Medical
  Branch
Galveston, Texas 77550

Frank J. Vollert
Superintendent
Galveston Independent School
  District
Galveston, Texas 77550

Mildred Vorsburgh
Home Counselor—Family Plan-
  ning
Galveston County Community Ac-
  tion Council
Galveston, Texas 77550

Barbara E. Williams
Director, Adolescent Inpatient
  Unit
Division of Child & Adolescent
  Psychiatry
The University of Texas Medical
  Branch
Galveston, Texas 77550

Jim Williams
Coordinator, Educational Plan-
  ning
The University of Texas Medical
  Branch
Galveston, Texas 77550

Mildred C. Williamson
Coordinator of Health Services
Galveston Independent School
  District
Galveston, Texas 77550

Christine Wright
Pediatric Resident
The University of Texas Medical
  Branch
Galveston, Texas 77550

Gregg F. Wright
Fellow in School Health
The University of Texas Medical
  Branch
Galveston, Texas 77550

Anita Yanes
Home-School Agent
Galveston Independent School District
Galveston, Texas 77550

Eli Douglas
Superintendent
Garland Independent School District
720 Stadium
Garland, Texas 75040

Betty A. Williams
Coordinator Health Services
Garland Independent School District
720 Stadium
Garland, Texas 75040

Andres E. Chavez, Jr.
Alderman—City of Hidalgo
Box 55
Hidalgo, Texas 78557

Esther C. Chavez
Interested Citizen/Teacher
P.O. Box 155
Hidalgo, Texas 78557

Bertha C. Garcia
Assistant Principal
Hidalgo Independent School District
P.O. Drawer D
Hidalgo, Texas 78557

Fred G. Garcia
Superintendent
Hidalgo Independent School District
P.O. Drawer D
Hidalgo, Texas 78557

Norma L. Garza
Teacher
Hidalgo Independent School District
P.O. Drawer D
Hidalgo, Texas 78557

Luz Pezzat
Community Health Aide
P.O. Box 479
Hidalgo, Texas 78557

Joel Rodriguez
City Commissioner
P.O. Box 705
Hidalgo, Texas 78557

Eduardo C. Vela
Mayor, City of Hidalgo
Box 187
Hidalgo, Texas 78557

Evangeline D. Vela
Interested Citizen/Teacher
Box 187
Hidalgo, Texas 78557

Vilma T. Falck
Director of Health Education
University of Texas Health Science Center
P.O. Box 20367
Houston, Texas 77025

Martha Licata
Nurse Consultant
Harris County Department of Education
6208 Irvington Blvd.
Houston, Texas 77022

Dorothy T. Schultz
School Health Consultant
Catholic Schools of Galveston-Houston
1700 San Jacinto
Houston, Texas 77002

Virginia Thompson
Director, School Health Department
Houston Independent School District
3830 Richmond
Houston, Texas 77027

Armin D. Weinberg
Baylor College of Medicine
Houston, Texas 77030

Ruth M. Cady
Professor/Coordinator Allied Health
Sam Houston State University
Huntsville, Texas 77340

Mary R. Sheehan
Coordinator Pupil Appraisal
Clear Creek Schools
League City, Texas 77573

James W. Caldwell
Pediatrician
600 S. Broadway
McAllen, Texas 78501

Jim Crow
Executive Director
Permian Basin Rehabilitation Center
512 E. 13th
Odessa, Texas 79761

Keith Dial
Director Special Education
Ector County Independent School District
Box 3912
Odessa, Texas 79760

Charles B. Lambeth
Pediatrician
1500 Westbrook
Odessa, Texas 79761

Betty Langston
School Nurse
Ector County Independent School District
Box 3912
Odessa, Texas 79760

J. M. Lilly
Public Information Supervisor
Ector County Independent School District
Box 3912
Odessa, Texas 79760

Oleta Phillips
Supervisor, Office of Elementary Education
Ector County Independent School District
Box 3912
Odessa, Texas 79760

Harley D. Reeves
Health Planner
Permian Basin Regional Planning Commission
P.O. Box 6391
Odessa, Texas 79762

Gail Smith
Director of Secondary Education
Ector County Independent School District
Box 3912
Odessa, Texas 79760

Hector Hugo Gonzalez
Representative—National League for Nursing
Chairman, Nursing Department
San Antonio College
San Antonio, Texas 78212

Jerry Newton
Director, School Health Services
San Antonio Independent School
  District
San Antonio, Texas 78205

Ora Prattes
Executive Director
Barrio Comprehensive Child
  Health Care Center
1102 Barclay
San Antonio, Texas 78207

Marietta Crowder
Director, Tyler-Smith County
  Health Department
Rt. 7—Box 150
Tyler, Texas 75707

Utah

Marshall Kreuter
College of Health
University of Utah
Salt Lake City, Utah 84112

Robert Louis Walker
Granite School District
Salt Lake City, Utah 84115

Vermont

Nina T. Cathcart
Pediatric Nurse Practitioner
9 Belmont Ave.
Brattleboro, Vermont 05301

John Y. Trumper
School Physician
9 Belmont Ave.
Battleboro, Vermont 05301

Washington

Elizabeth Bryan
School Physician
Edmonds School District
8500 200th SW
Edmonds, Washington 98020

Michael Warden
Director of Special Education
Edmonds School District
8500 200th SW
Edmonds, Washington 98020

Eleanor Dudley
Health Consultant—Special
  Education
Kent Public School
Kent, Washington 98031

Vivian K. Harlin
Director of Health Services
Seattle Public Schools
815 4th Ave.
Seattle, Washington 98109

Index